Praise for Shawn Paulsen

Sometimes our toughest times provide us with highlights of our lives. I moved to Utah in 2001 to take a radio job, and I didn't know a soul. It was a big risk, but without risk in life there is no reward. It turned out to be one of the biggest disasters of a life filled with them, but a highlight was meeting my friend Shawn Paulsen. Little did I know he was going through a whole mountain of problems of his own, as many of us do without mentioning them.

As a professional entertainer, it's not often that I call a club owner "friend" over business contact. Shawn was a rare exception and we became good friends that lasted past his comedy club and my radio job. He and his family are "real", and I grew to love and admire them all. Learning of Shawn's rare condition made me cry, but his unbelievable courage in the face of such a daunting challenge is inspiring beyond words. He is a true "mentsch" as the Jewish people call it. He walks tall and proud, but remains approachable and humble. I am proud to call him my friend, and would do anything and everything within my power to support anything he does. Keep slugging buddy! I know you've got more left in the tank.

—Dobie Maxwell Comedian /Author of Monkey in the Middle

Why Not Me?

Patty -

Always live for the moment. Never give up. You got this

[signature]

Why Not Me?

Choosing to be Positive in the Face of Adversity

A Memoir of Fear, Trust and Illness

Shawn Paulsen

AUTHOR ACADEMY elite

WHY NOT ME?
Copyright © 2016 Shawn Paulsen
All rights reserved.

Printed in the United States of America

Published by Author Academy Elite
P.O. Box 43, Powell, OH 43035
www.AuthorAcademyElite.com

All rights reserved. No part of this publication may be reproduced, stored in a retrieval system, or transmitted in any form or by any means—for example, electronic, photocopy, recording—without the prior written permission of the publisher. The only exception is brief quotations in printed reviews.

The author and the publisher have made every effort to ensure that the information in this book is correct. The events, locales, and conversations are based on the author's memories of them. Some names and identifying details have been changed to protect the privacy of individuals.

Paperback ISBN: 978-1-943526-93-2
Hardcover ISBN: 978-1-943526-92-5

Library of Congress Control Number: 2016914897
Author Academy Elite, Powell, OH

For my children:
Tyler (Kid) & Taylee, Arandalyn (Little One) & Justin.
For my grandchildren and great-grandchildren:
Bug & Skyler
Little Man
Pooh Bear
Happy Meal
Kamāmā
Brick
MJ
Tiny Might
You are my light in the darkness.

Contents

Introduction xv

Part 1: Why Me

1. Don't Blink 3
2. Bigger Is Not Always Better 12
3. To The Left 21
4. From Cancer To Syphilis 27
5. Blindsight 38
6. Speak Up 46

Part 2: The Old Me

7. Skating On Milk 55
8. I Am Iron Man 63
9. Dr. Jekyll And Mr. Hyde 69
10. Mom Said I Would Never See 13 78
11. I Punched Him Sober 86
12. Time To Be A Man 94
13. Saved By An Angel 100

Part 3: The New Me

14. A New Family 117
15. And Then There Were Four 121

16. Cops And Robbers........................... 132
17. It's All Downhill From Here..................... 140
18. Make Me Laugh............................ 150
19. It Wasn't Me 160
20. Mothers And Sons.......................... 166
21. Planes Trains And Automobiles 174
22. Mistakes 181
23. Go Straight To Grandkids 190

Part 4: Why Not Me

24. Too Dumb To Be Afraid...................... 199
25. Dogs Are The Best Medicine 207
26. Lost But Not Forgotten 219
27. The Song Of The Loon 226
28. Dis-Ability................................ 232
29. Can I Get A Spot........................... 241
30. Blind Luck................................ 247
31. Mr. Heat Miser 257
32. Overcome With Laughter..................... 265
33. Why Not Me.............................. 274

About The Author 279

Acknowledgements

Through all the hardships in my life, this book has been the most difficult thing I've ever done. It took 48 years of my life to compile these memories and trials. I have dedicated a year and a half to the completion of this memoir. Being mostly blind created its own issues with writing, and I struggled with an overwhelming desire to give up. I do not give up easily, and this hurdle is a testament to desire and courage.

The pitfalls and frustrations were much more difficult than I anticipated. Although the words and stories of this book flowed from me like a waterfall—writing as much as four to ten thousand words a day—the voice to text program that I used created its own ideas. Sentences like, *"Jesus eats pizza with the Eagles."* Sure, the Eagles are a great band and maybe Jesus likes their music, but I have no idea why or how it ended up in the manuscript. What took me three months to put on paper took eight months of rewriting.

I would not have been able to achieve this goal without the help of people who were willing to sacrifice to assist me in its completion.

Kary Oberbrunner, you gave me the opportunity to publish my story. You believed in me and mentored me through the demanding details of publishing.

Lisa Wood Bingham, thank you for taking what I call the English language and actually making it readable and understandable. I am eternally grateful to you and your incredible talent with words. You have been honest and helpful during this entire process. Although I have spent my life telling stories and performing on stage, you taught me that having a story to tell isn't enough.

My life has always been private, and to share it with others is a scary proposition, to say the least. Sara Walker, Nancy Rolfe, Melissa Beyer, Curtis Kidd, and Taylor Nelson, because of your insights and honesty, your wisdom and thoughts, this was much easier and more beneficial. You gave me the will to allow my story to be published.

My wife, children and grandchildren, you stood by me and supported all of my adventures. My parents and sisters, we may not always get along and don't get to see each other as much as we should, but you are always in my heart and I love each of you.

Uncle Roy and Aunt Carol thank you for all the years of support and continued involvement in my life. You have both been there through the good and bad times, and have had a greater impact on me than you know.

Kim Palmer, when my life changed drastically with this disorder, I was in a very dark and lonely place. You spent hours beyond measure helping me to understand my new life and dealing with the emotional issues that I faced. You became a close and trusted friend as well as a confidant. You enabled me to realize that my life was good enough and I didn't need to pretend to be anything else.

Last, and most important, my fans, followers and friends; you are the reason I continue. My shows are a product of your laughter and encouragement. It's because of you that I have the desire to press forward and test the limits of my disorder. Your unwavering support has inspired me to believe in myself and my real accomplishments, and not hold on to fantasies from my make-believe world.

"We all have two lives. The second one begins when you realize you only have one."

— *Confucius*

Introduction

"My body sometimes feels sore, but it works. I don't sleep well most nights, but I do wake up to fight another day. My wallet is not full but my stomach is. I don't have all the things I ever wanted but I do have everything I will ever need. I'm thankful because although my life is by no means perfect, it's my life and I'm happy"

— *Unknown*

It's a beautiful late spring day in May. The sun is shining and there is a slight cool breeze in the air. It's one of those days that, after the long dreary winter, makes you want to forget about work or any other plans you may have made, and just go to the nearest park to lay on the grass, allowing the sun to warm your body. After all, it has been neglected for far too many winter months.

You can smell the freshly blooming flowers and hear the birds gathering materials for their nests in preparation for the arrival of their soon-to-be family. White, puffy clouds are drifting by as if they don't have a care in the world. You know they mean no harm so you relax completely.

So here I am, lying on my back, listening to classic rock. However, it's not clouds, or birds I see, nor is the sun warming my body. But rather, I'm staring straight up at the gray-white plastic ceiling that looms above my head, trying not to hear the metallic grinding, clicking and humming that I am all too familiar with by now. Between that and the chill in the room, I long for the grass in the park even more.

I am into my second hour of a three and a half hour long MRI. The coffin-like chamber is poorly designed for a human—let alone a full grown man—and to be there for three and a half hours is unbearable. My shoulders ache and my ears ring from the noise of the test, even over the music that is playing in my headphones. I was told it would only be 45-minutes, but somewhere in that time, my doctor called and asked for further studies.

I've been seeing a group of eye specialists at one of the leading eye centers in the country. At this moment, they're as much in the dark about what is happening to me as I am. I have been oddly and abnormally losing my eyesight. Right now, the lower half of the vision in my left eye is gone, and it has progressed to the central vision of my right eye. The specialists working on my case can't for the life of them determine why. And they've never seen anything like it.

This scares me to death.
I'm going blind.

The past five weeks have been an absolute nightmare for me. Not just the kind that wakes you up at night in a cold sweat, but the kind that doesn't stop when you wake up. This is not new to me. When I sleep, my nightmares are reliving my childhood—the abuse and mental dissection that I went through with my father—the physical beatings that left me bruised and broken occurred almost weekly. I was always being punished for his mistakes, not with a 'time out' but with a closed fist.

The past that I thought I had discarded has now lifted its ugly head and, like a chimera, reminds me that even though I'm an adult and have accomplished so much in my life that I should be proud of, I still feel worthless. It was beaten into me both physically and emotionally by the one person who was supposed to be there to raise and support me.

Now, my nightmare continues even after I wake. I'm missing all of those beautiful things that I was accustomed to seeing every morning, welcoming me as the sleep cleared from my eyes. Not knowing if I am awake or asleep, it's as if somewhere in my mind, I have finally cracked, and I can no longer tell reality from fantasy. When I awake, the darkness sets in. I feel my eyelids open and close, the scene only slightly changing. From complete darkness to the shadows and blurred light that is now my vision. I know that my eyes are open, but in some way, they feel as if they are still closed. The once bright and sharp images are now dull and ghostly.

Every morning there is a civil war in my head, as the conscious and unconscious fight over the new reality that is mine. The rising sun that I used to greet with loving arms now brings an uncomfortable sensitivity. Heart disease and stroke-like symptoms affect my daily activities, and sometimes even getting out of bed is more than I can handle. The ache in my muscles and the weakness in my body are a constant reminder that I'm alive and moving under the control of something that's beyond me…it is a stranger to me…a stranger that will soon become my closest companion.

—Darwin's Evil Twin—

I believe all of these troubles have prepared me for the biggest challenges of my life. The abuse I suffered was far beyond what discipline or punishment should be. I would overcome this and move on to become proficient in various fields including law enforcement, entertainment, and therapy. I would marry my high school sweetheart and raise a family. Working extremely hard, I'd receive a Ph.D. and start several successful businesses. My struggles would be compounded by falling down a mountainside, being electrocuted, and nearly drowning, sustaining physical and mental injuries. Time after time I have been on the precipice of stupidity that should have ended in death. Yet here I am, still alive to tell the stories.

Recently I have realized that an education doesn't always come from books or structured classes. My views have changed over the past few years. I understand now that it is my life's experiences, failures, misfortunes, and disappointments that have made me the person that I am today. I still believe in education, and I still continue to study and learn but I place more value in my experiences.

My point is, you need to live for the moment and not pass up opportunities. At this time, I realize that I have only 'NOW' to accomplish what I want in life. I don't have the luxury of procrastination. I understand that my time is greater than any monetary items. The time I have with my family and enjoying the places that I love are most important.

You may be familiar with Darwin's Theory of Evolution. It is a notion that all life is related and has descended from a common ancestor. Darwin's general theory presumes that complex creatures evolve from more simplistic ancestors naturally over time. As random genetic mutations occur within an organism's genetic code, the beneficial mutations are preserved because they aid survival—a process he coined as 'natural selection.' These favorable mutations are passed on to the next generation. Over time, favorable mutations are kept, and the result is an entirely different organism, not just a variation of the original, but an entirely different creature.

For example, let's say a member of a species developed a functional advantage; i.e. grew legs and learned to walk. The new enhanced offspring would inherit that advantage and pass it on to their offspring and so on. The original members of the same species would gradually die out, leaving only the superior or advantaged members of the species.

I am proof that 'natural selection' is not always perfect; those genetic mutations aren't always a benefit to future generations. Sometimes those genetic mutations are flaws that create disorder and disease, and they, too, can be passed from generation to generation. These harmful genetic mutations generally mean that the individual will eventually die out. However, in my case, not before

INTRODUCTION

I can make a mark in this world and help others understand that time is short and life is precious and fragile.

It is imperative to make every moment count, never give up and always believe that there's something better. I thought that the symptoms of this disease were the end of my life, but I have learned it is just the beginning. My life has dramatically changed, but I've come to love, live, and enjoy life more than ever before.

I now get to see my existence in a whole new light—through the darkness. I'm experiencing things in a way that I know I never could have, had this disease not affected me. I seem to understand and realize more about what's going on around me. I have always lived, by necessity, in my make-believe world. It was my way of escaping the negative realities of my childhood. Because of this disease, I've learned to live my life with a couple of new mottos or beliefs. The first, *'Live for the moment.'*

Every minute in this life is worth living, whether you're at work, with family, or even in the presence of people that you don't want to be around. Every moment is worthwhile and has something to cherish because, in the blink of an eye, everything can change and those moments will become more precious to you than ever before. My other motto is, *'Attempt everything in life as if you cannot fail.'* Imagine what you could accomplish in your lifetime if you believed you could not fail.

What would you start?

In the following chapters you will get an in-depth look into my life. Some of the stories and events have never been told before. It is not intended to create pity or to assault the integrity of others, but to uplift and show that no matter what happens in life, we can still smile and carry on.

Part 1
Why Me

1
Don't Blink

"Do not confuse my bad days as a sign of weakness. Those are actually the days I am fighting my hardest."

— *Unknown*

There is a fifth dimension, beyond that which is known to man. It is a dimension as vast as space and as timeless as infinity. It is the middle ground between light and shadow, between science and superstition, and it lies between the pit of man's fears and the summit of his knowledge. This is the dimension of imagination. It is an area which we call the Twilight Zone.

— *Rod Serling*

The Twilight Zone was a science-fiction television series created by Rod Serling. The series depicted stories of paranormal, futuristic, or otherwise disturbing or unusual events. Each story typically featured a moral and a surprise ending. This is how I feel living day to day, lost somewhere between reality and a marionette in a sadistic puppet show, being controlled by some outside force that enjoys watching me squirm. It's the easiest way to express my life.

To help you understand, close your eyes almost entirely so that all you see is a slight amount of light and blurry shadows. Now condense that down in your mind to just a small dot. Visualize that the dot in your right eye is in the lower inside corner, closest to your nose, and that same small dot in your left eye is in the upper outer corner; the remaining visual field is dark gray to black. If you took the vision picture of my right eye and flipped it top to bottom, it would match my left eye perfectly. This is what my vision is like on a daily basis; the results of a maddening, spiraling, six-week block in time.

I went from 20/20 vision to a 90% vision loss in just six weeks, actually watching it disappear. Looking at something and seeing the darkness envelop it like something from an old black and white horror movie where the giant blob just continues to destroy and gobble up all the buildings and people in its path. However, with me, it was only gobbling up my vision, causing the people and things I grew so accustomed to seeing disappear like a terrifying magic trick.

The genetic markers are so obscure that intensive and painful tests would have to be done just to isolate the particular gene causing the problems. On top of all that, insurance would not pay for this type of testing, so it would all be out of pocket costs, which could run from tens to hundreds of thousands of dollars. Furthermore, the only benefit from this testing is the knowledge of which gene is the culprit. The treatment, or lack thereof, and the progression of the disease would not change. Add on top of all that, hearing loss, heart weakness, stroke-like episodes and complete and total muscle fatigue and constant burning and you get a pretty fair picture of what I go through.

For over a year, this phenomenon baffled doctors. Not just regular doctors, but specialists who are renowned as the best in their field. Ophthalmologists, neurologists, neuro-ophthalmologists, geneticists—you name the specialty, I've seen them, and they've seen me. The specialists could not figure out the reason for my vision loss and the exact inverse of vision and lack of sight in the right and left eyes. Even after years of testing, hospital stays, doctors, blood transfusions, treatments and so on, I've been told that there is no formal diagnosis for my disease.

My current specialist, who is world renowned for his work with this type of disease, is sure of the following things:

1. It is an energy failure disorder related to mitochondrial DNA. The closest disease is what's called Mitochondrial, Encephalomyopathy, Lactic Acidosis, and Stroke-like episodes, or M.E.L.A.S.
2. It is progressive, terminal, and there is no treatment or cure for the disease. Further testing wouldn't change anything.

Having a terminal illness with no definite timeline is like being stranded on a deserted island knowing that a rescue ship will be there July 15th and you've got to be ready, but you have no knowledge of what day it is. It's a constant reminder that this could be the day.

The greatest fear that I've had my entire life is losing my eyesight. I've always said that I could lose a limb, be paralyzed, or even lose my hearing, but I couldn't deal with losing my eyesight. Many people take their vision for granted—I know I did for a long time. It's one of those things that is always there, seeing the colors of the fall leaves, the faces of the people you love most, sunsets, stars, fireworks on the 4th of July—all of the things that we hold so dear and consider beautiful. I have always cherished my eyesight, and for the most part, it was always perfect.

Looking back now, I realize what a valuable tool my eyesight was. In most cases people don't think twice about their vision. It was always my eyes that, in a lot of circumstances, I relied on for survival; police work, hunting, everyday life.

When I was in my mid-twenties, my eyesight started to fail me. I went to an optometrist and, after a simple examination, got a prescription for glasses that corrected the problem. I never thought much of it, lots of people wear glasses and I would be one more. A few short years later, my eyesight seemed to be worse. I assumed I needed a new prescription but, to my surprise, the optometrist informed me that my vision was perfect and I no longer needed the glasses. He explained this was why I was struggling to see with them. We both found it quite strange that somehow my eyesight improved over the years and that my glasses were no longer necessary.

Little did I know that this would be a precursor to what was coming.

In April of 2014, I was traveling across the country on my annual Midwest run, performing for high schools during their all-night lockdown graduation parties. Earlier on, I used to fly to my first destination, rent a car, keep it for a month to drive to and from the shows, then fly home when needed. However, once I opened my clinic and needed to balance clients with out of state shows, this became too expensive, so I chose to drive instead of fly. Most of the drives were between 18 and 20 hours one direction.

I would leave early on Friday mornings and drive until late Friday night, find a hotel and then drive into the city where I was performing on Saturday, usually arriving with just enough time to check into the hotel and get a couple of extra hours sleep before my show. After performing, I would sleep for a couple more hours and then repeat the process back home.

I had traveled this way many times, but it was beginning to tire me and was hard on my body. I didn't know that I had an energy failure disorder, and couldn't understand why I hurt so badly after these long drives, or why I had such a hard time recuperating during the week, so I continued on. It was during this Midwest trip that I realized I had a blurry dark spot in my left eye. I thought I had scratched it, or maybe I had something in my eye. It wasn't necessarily in my vision, in fact, it was in the lower left-hand corner of my left eye, and it wasn't anything that concerned me at the time.

After returning home from that first trip, I went back to work at the clinic and realized the spot never went away. The next week's travel came and went, and it seemed that the spot had grown bigger.

Now it was starting to bother me; I was getting aches behind my eyes and the vision in that area was turning black.

Up until this point in my life, I had only experienced a handful of headaches; I felt pretty lucky because I've seen my wife deal with painful headaches our entire marriage and it was certainly nothing I wanted to experience. A few years before recognizing the start of this disease I experienced my first migraine. I remembered I was on my way home from a hunting trip with my father in law, and in just a few short minutes, I went from feeling fantastic to being in some of the most intense pain I've ever had in my life.

That short trip home seemed like an eternity to me. Every bump in the road, every time we turned or stopped, was like getting hit in the head with a tank. My father-in-law rushed me home as quickly as he could; making that 2-hour drive in just over an hour. When I arrived home, my wife wanted to rush me up to the hospital but I refused as always, and it finally went away. That was also the last migraine I ever experienced until this disease progressed further.

It was after the third trip to the Midwest that my eyes played a real trick on me. I began to have flashes or sparkling in my left eye. When I returned home, I told my wife that I needed to make an appointment with an optometrist. On April 29th, I went into the appointment totally unaware of what I was about to learn. I explained my situation to the optometrist, and he started a series of test, beginning with fundus photography.

If you've ever been to an optometrist before, you may have had this particular test. A high definition camera takes a picture using an extremely bright light that shines through the pupil and captures a clear image of the back of your eye. You get an incredible view of the inside of your eye.

After the photograph, the doctor immediately took me into a separate room and pulled them up on his computer.

He brought up the right eye first. Because of my schooling, I had some familiarity with the anatomy of an eye, so I understood what I saw. The optic disc (nerve bundle attachment) looks like a ping pong ball that has been cut in half, with a wet paper towel laid on top of it. It has a very crisp, perfectly round, sharp edge and looks like it is pressed against the eye. He then brought up my left eye. Before he could even say a word, I immediately spoke up, *"That's fucked up!"*

I'm not a medical doctor, but I could see that there was a problem. Where the optic disc attached to the back of my eye, it looked like a big white puffy cloud, like the ones you see floating by before a summer storm. It also looked as if somebody had taken my ping pong ball and smashed it, leaving jagged open edges all the way around.

He made a phone call to a local Ophthalmologist and electronically sent the photos and results of this exam to him. An Ophthalmologist is a Medical Doctor that specializes in the eye. The Ophthalmologist was quite concerned with the results of the photography and requested I immediately come to his office. I called my wife at work on my way to the appointment, picked her up and we went together. It was a short drive from her place of employment to the eye center, but in those 5 minutes, she and I discussed a whole realm of possibilities, including cancer.

I checked in at the receptionist desk, and was immediately escorted into an examination room. After a slew of new tests, the doctor believed I had a condition known as Anterior Ischemic Optic Neuritis, characterized by an inflammation of the optic nerve and, he believed, brought on by a T.I.A. I suffered earlier. (We cover T.I.A. in a later chapter.) He felt that it would go away naturally, and my vision would return, but wanted further testing.

I was scheduled to come back on May 6th. We went through more advanced tests and with the results, he felt that the Optic Neuritis had peaked and was now going to heal. Throughout the next week, between the 12th and 18th, the blind spot grew bigger. In fact, it started to cloud the entire lower portion of the visual field in my left eye. It was now progressing to my right eye, and the photopsia (those little sparkles of light I mentioned) was getting worse. It went from sparkles to fireworks. I had a gut feeling, the ones you don't ignore, and I knew at this point that it wasn't going to get better.

I contacted the Ophthalmologist for the third time and explained that it had progressed to my right eye, and I was in his office the very next day. It was now May 20th. After another hour of tests, the doctor decided it was time to refer me to the University Of Utah Moran Eye Center. He explained he had never seen anything like this and believed it was something beyond his scope of training and wanted their team of specialists to look at me.

To be seen at the Moran Eye Center you have to be referred by a doctor, and only a small number of referrals get accepted. It is one of the top eye centers in the country and has some of the most incredible doctors I've ever met in my entire life. My referral was immediately accepted, and I had an appointment with a Neuro-Ophthalmologist the very next day.

When the clinic confirmed my appointment, they told me to prepare for a long day; I would most likely be there for four hours. My wife took the day off, and we arrived at the Moran at 1:00 p.m. We left that day, utterly exhausted, at 6:30 p.m.

Many disorders and diseases that affect the brain produce visual symptoms. A Neuro-Ophthalmologist was assigned to me and she was at my side nearly the entire time. With training in both Neurology and Ophthalmology, these doctors work to diagnose and treat visual problems that arise from the nervous system as well as the eyes themselves. Not surprisingly they are sometimes difficult to diagnose. I spent the better part of three and a half hours, going from test to test involving my eyes, the optic nerves, and my brain itself. After the tests, I met with Doctor Croft.

I am not a very religious man, never have been, but I will say that Doctor Croft is an angel sent straight from God. From the moment that she walked into my room, she was warm and compassionate. She described everything that she wanted to do in high detail, and she involved me in every discussion and decision made. Even as my eyesight further diminished over time, she was always there for me. She would call me personally several times a week just to check up on me.

If she had any new information or ideas, she called me immediately to discuss them with me. She knew of my education and background, and she always talked to me as a colleague rather than a patient. At one point she gave me her personal cell number so I could get in touch with her if there were any changes. Doctor Croft's genuine concern will always be a glimmer of light in my darkness.

I must admit that every doctor and technician we came into contact were amazing and gifted people. I was always made to feel welcome and cared for by the entire staff. There never was, nor is, a moment that I didn't believe they had my best interest at heart.

As I progressed through the testing, I continued to travel and perform. However, it was a bit more difficult. Flash forward to that sunny spring day in May. As I lay in that M.R.I. tube staring at the cold gray ceiling over me, I watched as my right eye turned to near complete darkness. The only way for me to describe it is like someone injected black ink into my vision. As the ink swirled and darkened in my eye, I knew that there was no going back.

I am going blind.

When the test was over, the darkness had covered the entire upper right side and down through the central portion of my vision. My left eye had already lost the sight in the lower portion. As I left the hospital, I realized I had no business driving. My vision was so blurry and obscured that I was a danger to other drivers. I drove myself home and parked my truck, knowing that was it. I have not driven, with one exception, ever again.

The loss of driving after spending a lifetime doing it is indescribable. I have never felt so helpless, lost and stuck. I can no longer run up to the local mart just to grab that gallon of milk we need, or attend a doctor appointment without someone taking me.

I used to jump into my truck and go anywhere I wanted; drive a few hours to go fishing or just to clear my head. At times, it was my solace, my therapy. Now, I have permanent residency in the passenger seat. The luxury of driving is one that I will forever miss.

This is the most recent in the series of Twilight Zone episodes that is my life. After the long discussions with the specialist and following the sequence of symptoms in reverse, I realized that this wasn't the beginning of the disease; it was closer to the end. I hadn't realized it, but the symptoms had started years before, as early as elementary school, and had progressed throughout life. Fatigue, dizzy spells, lack of distinct memories—those were some of the previous manifestations. I had no idea what they would bring to pass.

> *"In the blink of an eye, your life can change due to disease. Your goals, dreams, and priorities are forced to take different turns. You are grateful for the little things and worry less about the big things. You leave behind the history of yesterday and determine how you will use today's energy. This is your life, and there is no time for drama."*
>
> — *Unknown*

I couldn't have said it better myself. At some point, we will all face a life-altering experience; whether it is the death of a loved one, a serious illness, or some loss that reminds us of what's most important. These experiences can teach us treasured lessons, help us discover inner strength, and realize what is truly important.

2

BIGGER IS NOT ALWAYS BETTER

"The gods envy us. They envy us because we are mortal, because any moment may be our last. Everything is more beautiful because we are doomed. You will never be lovelier than you are now. We will never be here again."

— *Iliad by Homer*

In 2010 I unknowingly experienced the first of the major symptoms of this disease. I was at my therapy clinic with a client when I started to feel some discomfort in my chest and pain radiating down my left arm. I also noticed that I was upset to my stomach and lightheaded. I've been through enough medical training to suspect that I was having a heart attack or some other type of heart issue. I have a difficult time asking for help or showing weakness, so I spent the remaining time with my client trying to ignore the symptoms and move through the therapy.

The symptoms were getting stronger, and I felt like if I didn't do something soon, I would probably lose consciousness. I pushed through it, as I always do, until my client's time was up, then I went home and rested for the remainder of the day. Yes, I know. But I'm pretty stubborn when it comes to doctors. I don't like to bother them when I feel like it's something that will pass. My wife got home, and the two of us decided it would be best if I was checked out. We went to an after-hours clinic instead of the ER, thinking that it could be acid reflux or a pinched nerve.

After spending several hours at the doctor's office and only a few tests and questions, the doctor concluded that he didn't believe I had a heart attack. He also thought it was probably stress related, or some other issue—maybe a pulled muscle. We returned home and I continued my day as normal. The next morning I felt much better, but was still a little lethargic and tired. Later that day, one of my good friends who is a physician contacted me and asked me if I wanted to go lunch with him.

Rod and I have been friends for 20 years, and he's been my personal physician through more than half of those. He has been part of this journey from the beginning, and there is no one I trust more. At lunch, I described my episode from the night before. He said that he didn't agree with the other doctor's diagnosis, and he wanted to be certain for himself. He had me come into his office the following day for a full exam.

As soon as I arrived, they were waiting for me, and I gave blood and a urine sample for typical standardized testing. He did a thorough exam, including chest X-rays and an E.K.G. There was an abnormality in the x-ray that he explained as hypertrophy, which is an enlarged heart. He contacted a cardiologist and, based on the X-ray, he believed further testing needed to be done as soon as possible to ensure there weren't any further problems. Rod made me an appointment with him in just a few short hours.

I was told by the Cardiology Department to wear loose clothing and to be at their office in two hours. When I arrived, they took me into a typical room—sterile, white and void of everything but the instruments and testing equipment which were to be used on my heart.

Most of the tests were relatively easy for me. All I needed to do was lay there and allow them to hook up the different devices to get the readings that they needed. They started with a more extensive electrocardiogram, where there are twice as many leads attached to my body than are used at the clinics.

This allowed them to get a much more definite and accurate reading. They also performed what is known as a bubble study to check for a possibility of a P.F.O., or Patent Foramen Ovale, which is a leak between the left and right sides of the heart.

Then came the echocardiograms. There are three of these tests performed in different ways. The first one is called a Transthoracic Echocardiogram; the standard echocardiogram which is similar to ultrasounds that pregnant women go through before birth. The second is a Doppler Echocardiogram this works the same way, but uses a different waveform. It allows the doctor to see the movement of the blood to make sure there are no obstructions or leakages. The last echocardiogram wasn't so easy or the least bit pleasant to experience.

As they were setting up the room for that third echocardiogram, I realized that two male technicians who each weighed between 230 and 250 pounds, also joined in on the fun. They brought with them a crash cart. For those of you not familiar with the medical field, a crash cart is a small metal cart that contains the necessary equipment to revive somebody if their heart should stop.

A second doctor entered the room as well. Now I'm laying in this room with two nurses, three technicians, two doctors and a crash cart thinking to myself, *"This is not going to be good."* I felt like I was in one of those 1960's cult war movies where they were going to torture information out of me and then make me disappear.

The doctor explained that they were going to do a stress echocardiogram. I don't do anything half-assed—I say *"Go big or go home,"*—and apparently the doctor had the same thoughts. His idea was to get my heart rate above 200 beats per minute. I'm no expert, but I do know that 200 beats per minute are a lot more than what is recommended. He told me that if I started to have any distress before that, they would stop the test and take measurements from there. However, he wanted to try and get it as close to that as possible.

At this point in my life, I believed that I was in pretty good shape. I had been active in martial arts and I hiked and hunted. Besides the heart issue, I felt pretty good. Little did I know how none of that was going to matter.

The first step was putting me on a treadmill. Not an ordinary treadmill, but one that monitors everything and does any speed. Like a Bionic Man, Barry Allen—A.K.A. The Flash—sort of treadmill. I stepped onto the treadmill, and the two large male techs strapped my hands down to the handles on each side. *"May I ask what the straps are for?"* I calmly said out loud, while internally it was, *"WHAT THE FUCK!"* They told me it was to keep me from falling off. Again, thinking to myself, *"If I were to fall off at that speed, wouldn't it yank my arms right out of the socket?"* However it was their test, and I was just here for the ride—literally.

They strapped a blood pressure cuff on my arm, and a monitor to my chest. I think it was so they would know if my heart stopped. The treadmill started up slowly to warm me up with a walk. My pulse climbed naturally and easily, starting in the mid 70's. About the time it hit the 120 mark, they injected me with some stimulant that caused my heart rate to accelerate very rapidly. In a matter of seconds, it climbed from 120 to 170 to 190 beats per minute. Now I have been through a lot of frightening things in my life. At times, I have stared them right in the face. But this?

This put all those times to shame.

I have never been afraid of much; I tell people all the time that I'm too stupid to be scared. It takes a smart man to be afraid of something and not push the edge of danger, but I have always dangled over the edge, held on with two fingers, and jumped in with both feet. But this scared the hell out of me.

In the time my heart rate went from 170 to 220 beats per minute, everything was a complete blur. My mind was racing, and I was far beyond worrying about how fast my heart was beating. I was going to die! I felt myself slip into my old world of anger and the fight or flight response kicked into full swing.

I did not like this feeling, and I wanted out. I was done with this test, the doctors and the instruments that brought me to this point. I will admit that I 'swear like a sailor' in my personal life, but I am usually very respectful around others. However, this day I started throwing the word *"FUCK"* around like it was the only thing left in my vocabulary. I called every person in that room every curse word I could muster. I threatened their lives, and I meant it.

I promised that doctor that as soon as he let me off the treadmill I was going to tear his heart out of his chest and show it to him so he could get a better understanding of how it worked. I have never been afraid to fight or to defend myself, and I believed that I was in that very situation. My flight response was broken, and my fight response was overactive.

It was at this time I learned what the two male technicians were for.

When my heart rate reached 220 beats per minute, the treadmill stopped. I was removed by the two male techs; it was their job to keep me from killing the doctor. Or so I imagined. In all reality, my heart rate was moving fast and they needed to get the ultrasounds and the pictures as quickly as possible. I was lifted off the machine and onto a table by the two men. There is an opening in the table where the side of my chest laid, and where the ultrasound transducer is. I realized that the doctors and techs had nothing to fear from me and my threats. Not because I was outnumbered or that the two techs outweighed me, but because of what occurred next.

I have never experienced this kind of testing in my life. Imagine the worst fear that you have and how it makes you feel, then times that by ten and you'd be close. The job of the two large techs was to hold me down onto that table. The stress that was applied to my heart and the adrenaline dump into my system caused my body to go into uncontrollable convulsions. It was their job to hold me as still as possible.

This was already difficult and I was panicking more than words can express. I didn't think it could get any worse, then the technician told me to hold my breath. She may as well have asked me to hold back the ocean's tide or push a mountain into the ground.

Between the techs holding my body still and the explanation that if they did not get the proper picture, we would be going through this again, I was suddenly convinced that I actually could hold my breath. I will say though, it was one of the most difficult things I've ever had to do in my life.

After two and a half hours of testing, I asked the Cardiologist about the crash cart. He nonchalantly stated, *"Just in case."* "Just in case what?" I asked. He replied, *"It's nothing to worry about. Just in case your heart stopped during the stress part of the exam."*

I'll admit I have endangered my life many times. I have placed myself in situations which, under normal circumstances, could have been very detrimental. But, they were *my* decisions. So I was a little bit irritated that he thought he had the right to place me in those same types of situations. I asked him what he would have done had my heart stopped, and he looked me right in the face, rather indifferently, and said with total confidence, *"I would have just brought you back."*

I do realize that these tests were necessary in order to get the correct information and to keep me as healthy as possible, but I was infuriated. Earlier I had noticed all of the different colored clothing that the people in the room were wearing to signify their different positions in the hospital. Dark blue for the nurses, gray for the techs and, of course, pristine white for the doctors. I always believed it was to show how clean and sterile everything was, but I now know it's because of the pillar that they think they stand on.

Apparently this doctor has replaced all of his pictures of God with mirrors. So I said, *"Nice to meet you, God!"* He did not appreciate me making a reference to the fact that he believed he had the power of life and death. He believed that as long as he was in that room, I had nothing to worry about.

Several days later I was contacted by the Cardiologist again. He wanted me to do one last stress test. I almost declined, remembering what the last stress test was like. However, he told me this one was much easier; it was *walking* on the treadmill, not *running*. He said that I had an appointment with Nuclear Medicine at 10:00 a.m. the next morning.

Nuclear Medicine is something that I am mildly familiar with. My Uncle Terry was the head of Nuclear Medicine and Radiology at this particular hospital when he was alive, and the person that is now running the N.M. portion of the hospital was trained by him. This made the test a lot easier because they were very close friends. We reminisced and laughed about all the good things and fun times with my uncle and how much we both missed him.

The test was easy to perform; before they started the actual test, they did a simple echocardiogram to determine a standard baseline of my heart at rest. After the first set of readings I once again stepped on a treadmill. However, this time, I was allowed to walk at a relatively quick pace.

Once my heart rate reached between 130 and 140 beats per minute—which is pretty standard with aerobic exercise—the nuclear technician came back into the room. He was carrying a cylinder about the size of a stackable chip can. But this chip can weighed about 40 pounds.

It was made out of pure lead to keep the radioactive material inside. This is where the panic set in. The technician was wearing a lead lined radioactive suit, gloves, and hood before he even opened this container. And here I was in shorts and a t-shirt walking on the treadmill in the middle of the room thinking to myself, *"Shouldn't I have some form of protection as well?"*

After the technician was fully armored and looking like an extra from the movie E.T., he opened the lid of the container and removed a small syringe. This reminded me of the bright green isotopes that are on The Simpsons during the beginning credits

BIGGER IS NOT ALWAYS BETTER

of the show. It was about the same size and shape, however it was clear and not the bright fluorescent glowing green. A bit of a letdown after what video games and movies have led us to believe.

However it was, indeed, radioactive and it was about to be injected into my bloodstream. I'm not a Nuclear Physicist, but I'm pretty sure this is not a procedure that is on the to-do list. After the injection, I was to continue walking on the treadmill for another five to ten minutes, and then they would do the echocardiogram once again.

He injected the radioactive isotopes and left the room, allowing me to microwave in peace. I continued my treadmill exercise for ten more minutes. I was then allowed to sit and relax, allowing my heart rate to come back down so that, once again, they could take pictures of my heart. The test provided images that might show areas of low blood flow through the heart and damaged heart muscle.

After all the testing had been completed, a second technician came into the room with release paperwork for me to sign because I had just been injected with radioactive materials. There was a lot of the typical medical jargon and disclaimers, but there was one statement that stood out in my mind—do not go to an airport or any military base.

This was very disconcerting to me. I loved to fly, both recreationally and as a necessity in my current career. Also, I lived just a few short miles from the Air Force Base, which didn't settle with me, either. I asked why that would be an issue. They told me it would set off their bomb detectors.

Apparently, if I were to go through the detectors at the airport or the gate at the Air Force Base, they are equipped with Geiger counters to make sure nobody is carrying radioactive material or any bombs onto the airplanes or the base. And I was currently a radioactive material!

This was not explained to me before this test. Although I had no plans to visit an airport or the Air Force Base at this particular moment, it was something that I did on a regular basis. I asked how long it would be before I could go back to the airport or the base and they said to be safe, two or three months. Which means I was right in visualizing the Simpsons. For two or three months, I would walk around like Homer Simpson glowing in the dark.

In the end, I was diagnosed with Hypertrophic Cardiomyopathy. Hypertrophy means that my heart is continuing to grow inside of my chest; for an unknown reason, the walls of my heart continue to increase. Cardiomyopathy simply means that the muscle itself is weak.

If you were to take a chest X-ray, you would see that an average person's heart is about the size of a closed fist. Mine is larger than my open hand. Not only is the heart larger, but the walls of the heart, or myocardium itself, is growing thicker. Which means the blood-pumping chambers of the heart are becoming smaller. It takes a lot more effort for my heart to pump the blood through my body and it pumps less than my body requires.

This was one of the reasons I became weak so quickly and that the lactic acidosis in my muscles was so high. My heart was a weak muscle working twice as hard to pump a fraction of the blood that was necessary for my body.

3

TO THE LEFT

*"No matter how hard your life is,
go to bed grateful you still have one.*

— *Unknown*

I had been struggling on and off with my heart condition for four years. At times, weeks or months would go by, and I wouldn't feel a single symptom. Then other times, I couldn't go an entire week without having some chest pain or syncopal episode. One particular morning, In February of 2014, I was walking through a major chain store in the dog food aisle.

It was about 10:00 a.m., and before I knew what had happened, I found myself sitting on top of the bags of dog food, coming to terms with the massive pain in my chest. When I looked up, my wife was standing over me with an incredibly concerned look on her face trying to get me back to awareness. This was by far the worst chest pain I had experienced up to this point.

After a few moments, the pain started to subside, and I could breathe a little better. As usual during these episodes, I immediately chewed up and swallowed baby aspirin to help thin the blood and alleviate some of the symptoms of the pain and pressure in my chest. These episodes were becoming commonplace, and we had a system down. The unique thing about that day was that it was my wife's birthday, and although we hadn't made any significant plans, we had discussed doing a few things to celebrate. After the episode that morning, we decided it would be best just to go home and relax for a little while, then make a decision on what to do later that evening.

Often after one of these episodes I feel drained, and a lot of times the pain in my chest doesn't go away for several hours or can even last all day. But that evening, after several hours of relaxing at home, I started to feel better. I decided that I would be okay, and wanted to go to dinner with the rest of the family to celebrate.

At the restaurant, I was holding, cuddling and playing with my grandchildren, laughing and joking, as always. As a side note, *'as always'* is a familiar phrase. I constantly have the pain and the feeling of discomfort and fatigue. I've made sure that throughout this entire disability, no matter what pain I happen to be in, people see me 'as always' happy, laughing and joking. There are very few people whom I let into that inner circle of how I feel and what is really going on.

When I try to explain to people what it's like, all I can say is that I feel *'Off'* or *'Different'*. I do not have the words to describe the feeling that I get as my body shuts down. I frequently get asked to describe it, *"What do you mean you don't feel well?" "Are you sick to your stomach, have a headache, does something hurt?"* I don't have a way to explain what it feels like—a particular sense or dysfunction—all I can say is, *"I don't feel well."*

I've had to tell my family that's the only explanation that I have and please don't ask me further questions, because I don't have those answers. I know that it is just as difficult, disheartening and frustrating for them to hear and try to understand as it is for me to attempt to explain.

Anyway, after we finished eating, my wife asked if we could return to the store to pick up some of the things that we didn't get earlier that day when I had my episode. I told her I was feeling much better and that I believed I would be okay. As we were walking through the store, I unconsciously started rubbing the left side of my face. I didn't even realize that I was doing this until we got to the checkout counter.

It was as if a lightbulb turned on and I realized that it was numb to the touch. I was having a terrible time forming words and making my jaw open and close correctly. As I was standing there rubbing the side of my face, my wife looked at me very puzzled and asked what I was doing? I told her that the left side of my face was numb.

My wife was a 911 dispatcher for 15 years and had dealt with this type of situation repeatedly. She realized some of the symptoms that I was having, and she immediately went into evaluation mode.

"Lift your arms?"
"Smile."
"What day is it?"

She realized I was having a hard time answering her questions and that it seemed as if I couldn't even form the words. I knew the answer, but the words just wouldn't come. She asked if I wanted an ambulance or if she should take me up to the hospital. Of course I'm stubborn as a mule, and even more so when it comes to hospitals. Even though I knew this was a serious situation, I opted to drive there.

As I got out of the car in the parking lot of the hospital, my wife noticed that I was dragging my left leg. She asked why I was limping, and I didn't have an answer for her. I just couldn't use my left leg. It felt like a water balloon—I don't know how else to explain it. She said I acted like it was weighted and it was difficult for me to pick it up.

As we entered the emergency room doors, I realized that the trip to the hospital was a blur. I didn't remember leaving the store, and somehow we were now at the hospital. Typically when going into an emergency room, you are directed to the intake area or desk where they process you to determine the priority of your emergency or how quickly you should be seen. In this particular case, a nurse met me right at the door. Or at least that's how I remember it.

I later asked my wife if she had called to tell them we were coming, or if she knew how the nurse knew to meet us. She said she had no idea what I was talking about, we entered and went to the admitting desk, and they called a nurse to take me right into a room for processing. I still don't recall that ever happening. What I do remember is the nurse had a very concerned look on her face.

At the time, I thought I said out loud, *"Why do you look so scared? You're a nurse?"* But apparently, that was never said and neither were answers to the other questions she was asking me. My wife later told me that I just kept looking at her with a very lost and puzzled look on my face as if asking for help answering the questions. All I can recall is that I couldn't figure out how to make the answer come out of my mouth.

The nurse set off an alarm to bring more doctors and nurses to my side as a possible stroke. From this moment until the following day, everything was a blur. I remember doctors and nurses coming in and out of the room and talking to me. However, I can't remember what they asked or what they were doing. The few questions I remember:

Doctor: "Do you know what day it is?"
Me: "My wife's birthday."
Doctor: "What date is your wife's birthday?"
Me: "It's my wife's birthday."

The most memorable aspect of this entire experience was the look on my wife's face. For the past four years, we had been dealing with my heart issue, and she had grown accustomed to that. This time, she had a look of panic and fear which I had not seen before.

By the time the initial evaluation was completed and I was being taken in to have a CT scan to check for hemorrhages or blood clots, the reflexes in my left arm and leg had diminished significantly. According to the doctor's report, the left side of my face had also reduced in movements such as smiling or being able to puff out my cheeks.

In a stroke, time is very critical; if left unattended too long it can cause irreversible damage and permanent paralysis. If treated quickly enough, some of that damage and paralysis can be alleviated. The doctor believed at the time that I had an Ischemic Stroke. This type of stroke is a blood clot rather than a rupture of a vessel. The prescribed treatment for an Ischemic Stroke is Tissue Plasminogen Activator or T.P.A.

This particular treatment dissolves the clot and reestablishes blood flow to the part of the brain that is deprived. The general rule is that it needs to be applied within three hours of the onset of the stroke to benefit the patient. From the initial onset of the numbness in my face until I was evaluated by the physician, only 45 minutes had passed, so we were well within this window. The doctor explained to us that if the T.P.A. is administered and it was not an Ischemic Stroke, it could be more detrimental and possibly fatal. After the CT scan and initial evaluation, he determined that we were safer to wait and not administer the T.P.A. I was admitted to the hospital for further evaluation and treatment by a neurologist.

I spent the next four days in the hospital and after a multitude of tests, the doctors were still confused. They had performed many of the typical tests that I've grown accustomed to—MRI's, blood work, and heart scans—but still no answers. On the plus side, this was the first time that I have had an electroencephalogram or E.E.G.

I was assigned to Physical Therapy and Occupational Therapy Departments to determine if my muscle weakness on the left side of my body was treatable. Their evaluation determined that the muscle weakness and lack of reflexes were apparent and that further therapy would be advised to regain use of my arm and leg once again. I was given several physical exercises to complete on a daily basis to try and speed up the process.

After all the testing and assessments, no one seemed to understand what was going on or why the left side of my body was displaying the symptoms. On the fourth day, the neurologist who was assigned to my case came to see me. He did a physical assessment to see my gate in walking and using my left arm.

The doctor took me out into the hallway, and we started walking. As we did, the typical dragging of my leg and weakness of my arm were very apparent. The doctor then started walking faster pulling me along with him until we were almost at a full run going down the hallway. I was frightened and stunned by this action; almost falling to the ground several times as I tried to drag my right leg up fast enough to catch myself from the failing left leg.

After the jog around the nurses station, the doctor and I spoke once again. He noted that my strength and ability to move increased with the added fear of falling or injury. This led him to believe that some of this symptomatology was psychosomatic in nature. He started to bring up things in my past that may have caused some of these issues to arise, and this is when I was suddenly flooded with scenes from my past. It was as if I had relived 10 years of my life in 30 seconds. It took me by surprise, and it was so shocking to my system that it was as if the stroke occurred all over again.

I felt as if my mind just would not function any longer and I was in a stupor. He was asking me questions that I knew the answers to, but I could not answer him. I was lost and confused. I felt like an eight year old child again trapped in a 45 year old body; running away and hiding from Mr. Hyde. After he left the room, I broke down and wept. Parts of my childhood were revealed to me that I didn't know existed. I had repressed them and hidden them away for so long that it was as if they hadn't occurred. But at that very moment, I was reminded that they had.

After being released from the hospital with no clear diagnosis and doctors still baffled by my symptoms, I spent six weeks in rehabilitation therapy to regain the use of my arm and leg. However the confusion and horror of the memories and thoughts in my mind we're not so easily dealt with.

4
From Cancer To Syphilis

> *"Every man takes the limits of his own field of vision for the limits of the world."*
>
> — *Arthur Schopenhauer*

By June, I was seeing Doctor Croft once a week. She was quite concerned about the rapid decline of my vision which made me the topic of discussion for the group of doctors at the Moran. The process that I was going through with testing and treatments was overwhelming but with my schooling and background, I understood most of what was being asked of me.

By this point the most common eye exam— *'Close one eye and read the chart on the wall'*—was useless. I could still see movement and, if close enough, I could make out objects but that was the extent of my vision. The 3-D vision, color chart and flicker test were stopped weeks ago. The flicker test is twelve different LEDs that flashed more rapidly as they progressed from one to twelve. Although I could still see light and dark, the problem with this test is that it used red lights. Sometime in the past few weeks I totally lost the ability to see red.

This was one more piece of the puzzle called my life; I have a form of colorblindness. My particular type is protanopia which means even in the small portion of vision that I have, I can't see red. When I tell people that red is invisible to me, for some reason people automatically believe that I have some superpower. I can't count the number of times I've been asked. *"If I had on a red shirt, would you be able to see through it?"* Depending on who is doing the asking, this may be a good thing to have. But it's not X-ray vision; it's just void of color.

Other tests showed the function of the rods and cones in the retina of my eyes. One test revealed that the vision loss was in my optic nerve and not in my eyes. In the doctor's words, *"Your eyes are gorgeous."* I don't mind saying that the physician reading the results from this particular exam was very attractive, and although I wished she were referring to my looks, I knew it was a reference to the anatomy of my eye. Still, It's pretty flattering to be told your eyes are gorgeous by a beautiful blonde, even if it is about their function and not the way they look on your face.

There was even a test where metal rings like contact lenses were attached to my eyes. For thirty minutes I stared at rapidly flashing colored lights in different and strange patterns. The connections measured the electrical impulses from my eyes. This test was the easiest of all of them. I didn't have to do anything; it was all up to the electrodes and patterns. After the test was over, I found out that it was designed not only to check the eye itself, but it was the only test that took out the patient's ability to influence it. This means that you cannot lie and say you are more blind than you actually are. When this test finished, I found out it showed I was more blind than I thought I was.

One of the most bizarre yet intriguing tests is fluorescein angiography. After an I.V. was established, I stared into a box void of all light. Several pictures of my eye were then taken to establish a baseline for the veins and structure of my eye. The fluorescein is injected into the I.V and from this point I cannot blink for several seconds. The camera takes pictures at a rate of one every second for twenty seconds. This determines how fast the chemical moves through the veins of the eye as well as locating any possible obstructions.

The bizarre part was after the test was over, everything was red—yes red!—the color I cannot see. The first time I was subjected to this test I still had some vision and lights, people, walls and everything were a different shade of red. This would go on for several minutes until my eyes would adjust and the colors would return…all except red.

Fun fact: fluorescein is eliminated through the urine. This wouldn't be an issue except that it glows a bright chartreuse green, and I mean green—picture a lightsaber from Star Wars glowing green—and it stains everything it touches. The first time I had this test, I was told this would occur and remain for several hours until it was eliminated from my system. I drank gallons of water to clean my system faster.

The second time I forgot about the glowing pee issue. We spent several hours at the Moran that day and by the time we left it was early evening, and we were hungry. We stopped at a local restaurant on the way home. I went into the restroom not thinking about the tests earlier that day. Even blind I could see what was happening in front of me, but it was too late to stop. As I finished my business, it appeared that I had painted the urinal with radioactive green.

I also learned that flushing repeatedly didn't change the soft glow that it produced. I was embarrassed and slightly amused as another man entered the restroom and stared curiously at the urinal before walking to the second urinal to relieve himself.

The other tests continued week after week; Attempting to track a dot of light in a dark circle; clicking buttons when I saw a small flash of light while looking straight ahead; looking at flashing colored panels, although not seeing them. This was the only way to track the progression of loss.

Besides all of the eye exams, they also required several blood exams. I was at the lab for blood draws every other week for some new diagnostic. Some of these tests were so rare and obscure, the lab technicians drawing my blood weren't entirely sure what to do. Some had to be flash-frozen while others had chemicals and other substances added to them before sending them off.

I tell everyone that I have been tested for everything from cancer to syphilis; which is a true statement, and the number of times I was tested is also beyond imagination. As an example, I was tested for Multiple Sclerosis six different times. This includes a high volume spinal tap or lumbar puncture. They stick a long needle into the lower part of the spine that allows the cerebral spinal fluid or C.S.F. to be extracted. In most cases they remove approximately twelve milliliters and test it for anything from M.S. to cancers. In my case, the first several extractions didn't produce anything. They wanted a broader picture, so they extracted between 30 to 40 milliliters.

For any of you who have had this procedure, you understand the tremendous pain that it induces via a migraine headache and flu-like symptoms. Needless to say, it's a miserable way to spend a day.

I was checked for any and all forms of cancers, even if there were no known eye issues associated with them. I was tested for most known autoimmune disorders that can cause blindness even if I didn't have any of the other symptoms. Graves, Usher Syndrome, Neuromyelitis Optica and the list goes on and on. They all came back negative.

Because there wasn't an apparent cause, the doctors decided to start treatments for autoimmune disorders to see if any changes occurred that could be linked to something specific. This began with intravenous steroids. These are not the metabolic muscle building steroids. These are the damaging cortical steroids.

The usual adult dose of Prednisone, which is a typically prescribed steroid, is 5 to 60 milligrams per day. I was infused with 1,000 milligrams per day for three days and then tapered down for the next six weeks to a negligible amount. There are too many side effects to try and list here, but a few were weight gain of 36 pounds in six weeks, facial and back acne, abnormally disturbing nightmares, and topping the list, uncontrollable anger.

I have spent most of my life trying to control my anger issues, which we'll discuss at length in later chapters. Thus, this was very troubling for me to have this problem reappear after working so hard to control it. And it wasn't typical anger either. This was *'Hulk-like'* anger with fits of destructive rage.

After this procedure didn't produce any positive results, Doctor Croft wanted to try something more aggressive. She wanted me to spend a week in the hospital, as she wanted tests and procedures performed that needed closer observation. However, during the time that she wanted me in the hospital, I had contract work in California.

I had already lost weeks of work and income due to this disease, and I had to make a decision. Should I fulfill those contracts so that I could pay my bills or go to the hospital to possibly alleviate losing any more of my vision?

I chose to continue with the contracts and go to California. At the time, it was a very tough decision, but looking back now it was the right one. At that point, it very easily could have been wrong. Deciding between a house payment and stopping the progression of the disease shouldn't be difficult. But I felt like my vision wasn't going to get better and having spent the last several months in and out of hospitals and the Moran Eye Center made it difficult for me to meet my obligations.

When I returned from California, I was admitted to the hospital for a week of assessment and treatments. The most important of these was plasmapheresis. It started with surgically inserting a large catheter in the jugular vein of the neck. It had three ports that extended from the neck; these attached to a machine that is, in essence, a big centrifuge. The machine takes all of the blood out of your system then spins it, separating the plasma, antibodies and other proteins from the blood.

Your blood, minus those removed elements, is then put back into your system. In this process, all of the antibodies in your system are completely removed. Those antibodies are what cause some autoimmune disorders.

After all of those are eliminated, your body will regenerate them naturally, bringing those antibodies and proteins back to a reasonable level. A small garbage bag sized container of plasma and antibodies were taken out of my body every day for seven days. This was several gallons of fluid.

After five days, I had to wait before finishing the final two days because my protein levels fell below the minimum standard. This was, without any doubt, the most painful experience of my life. I felt as if my entire body was flooded with acid and it was eating me from the inside out. I felt like I was in a furnace completely on fire, and my skin was melting off of my body. My eyes wanted to jump out of my skull; my ears started ringing so loudly I couldn't hear anything else. I started sweating profusely, my mouth started watering, and all I could think of was I wanted it to stop. I wanted the pain gone, and I didn't care how. I was on the 14th floor of the hospital, and they had to restrain me from diving out the window.

When the feelings started, I told the technician how I was feeling. By the time he could get help into my room; I was bent over the side of my bed holding onto my head with both hands. I felt like it was going to explode. There was a puddle of sweat on the floor below me large enough that it took a cleaning crew with a mop and a bucket to clean it up.

Between the technician and the nurses, they got me back into my bed and raised my feet to allow the blood to flow back to my head. It only took several seconds after that, and I started to regain my composure and my thoughts. The feelings of suicide, pain and claustrophobia dissipated rather quickly. Apparently, having a decreased amount of blood which was exacerbated by my heart condition, caused an adverse reaction within my body. For the next six treatments, I was inverted the entire time to ensure that this did not happen again.

The hardest part of this terrible experience was that this whole week of testing occurred over my birthday. My birthday has always been just another day and I have spent many of them working or traveling. At times, I've even forgotten it was my birthday. Other than a handful of occasions in my life, it's never been that important or something for which I took time to celebrate. But somehow, this time was different.

This wasn't just another day. This was the first birthday I experienced after losing my vision. I was nervous, scared and everything around me was crumbling and falling apart. I spent the day in the hospital with no one but nurses whose job it was to come in and check on me. As scared as I was, mostly I just felt so alone. All of these circumstances were difficult for me, but for some reason, it being my birthday made it even harder.

It all changed that evening when my entire family showed up—kids, grandkids, my wife and even my parents. They brought a cake and we all gathered in the hospital cafeteria. We ate dinner, shared cake and enjoyed each other's company. It was a very touching experience for me to have my entire family surrounding and supporting me, especially during one of the most painful and life-altering experiences I'd ever been through.

We spent several hours laughing together and enjoying that love that only a family can give. We walked outside and took pictures next to the fountain in front of the hospital, and even though my kids are the greatest gift I've ever received, they gave me something else—a large set of wind chimes. The chime tubes ranged from one and a half to five feet in length. They were deep and loud, and they still give me the most spectacular concerts ever.

After losing my eyesight, I realized how relaxing certain sounds were. Things that I never paid attention to before, I could listen to for hours on end. The sound of those wind chimes, to this day, is one of the most beautiful, relaxing things that I have ever experienced. The picture they draw in my mind as I listen is something that I can't describe.

I've always heard that when a person loses one sense, the others heighten and become more sensitive. And yes, I do think that I hear and smell things that others don't. People around me are constantly amazed at what I hear or smell that they were unaware of before I brought it to their attention. But it isn't that one sense compensates for the loss of the other. Rather, we allow some of our senses to become secondary to our vision.

Think of a dog; they rely on their sense of smell above their vision. It's their nose that they use to find their way or identify other dogs. Similarly, we rely on our eyes for the majority of our sensory input. When that is gone, we are made more aware of our other senses. They're not heightened necessarily, but just have the primary sensory input now. They no longer have to take a back seat to vision. It's not that I hear better now, I just pay more attention to it.

After being released from the hospital, Doctor Croft told me that there was no significant change or data. Everything that they had done up to this point had produced no information about my condition. I'd had eleven MRI's including the one that lasted three-and-a-half-hours, five CT scans, four high volume lumbar punctures, high doses of steroids and the removal of the antibodies in my system. All of which yielded *absolutely* no information or change.

What I did have was a list of things that weren't wrong with me. I knew that I was free of any forms of cancer, M.S., A.L.S., N.M.O., and a million other little acronyms had been ruled out. I also knew that I didn't have any forms of communicable diseases such as syphilis and gonorrhea, even all types influenza or colds that may have caused some of the symptoms were ruled out. According to my doctor, I was the healthiest person on this planet—who was going blind.

Still pursuing the possibility of it being an autoimmune disorder, I started a regime of replacing my antibodies. I had to go to the hospital once a week for four weeks where I would spend a day with an I.V. infusion of fresh antibodies called Immunoglobulins. I referred to these as immuno-goblins because I have a tough time saying immunoglobulins. I could just envision these tiny little goblins running around in my system killing off any of the viruses or other issues that could be causing my blindness.

An infusion process took several hours and by several hours I mean most of my day. I would show up at the hospital early in the morning, and they would start with an IV. A new bottle of antibodies was attached every two hours for six hours; finishing up with a standard saline bag to help hydrate me after sitting for all that time in hopes of alleviating some of the ancillary symptoms that the infusion created.

There were many side effects to this, including migraines and the feeling of sinus pressure. The worst side effect was for three days afterward feeling like you had the flu. And I mean the down in bed, aching joints, fever, and headache, and there's no way to stop it or relieve the symptoms flu.

There was nothing they could do to avoid this. It was just part of the process. Once a week for four weeks I would go in and get new immuno-goblins, and this flu would start over. After the initial first four weeks, I went every other week for the next month and then once a month for ten following months. For an entire year, I had the flu for one to two weeks out of every month.

Test after test, procedure after procedure, nothing changed. My eyesight continued to darken; the blackout episodes were increasing in frequency and my doctors were out of ideas; and now I was also starting to lose my hearing. I had seen four different specialists, from macular degeneration to forms of retinal disorders, cancer specialists to neurologists and all of them were utterly baffled—all were at a loss.

I continued to be seen at the Moran even though the tests results remained the same. We were all hoping that there would be some breakthrough. But, if nothing else, maybe I could be an example to somebody else. Maybe I could be the subject of learning for the doctors. I was given the opportunity to see the world in a whole new way, and I was determined to share that way with others.

A well-known and highly respected physician was scheduled to speak at the Moran. He was a pioneer in eye related diseases and treatments and the doctors at the Moran were excited to get a chance to hear him speak. Doctors from around the country were coming to attend this event in hopes of learning some new techniques and procedures from this medical practitioner. The doctors at the Moran asked him if he would be willing to look over my case and examine me to see if he had any insights into my disorder.

What ultimately happened was, not only the speaking physician, but also the dozens of other attending physicians reviewed my case. What a great honor for me to have this many physicians in one place—hundreds of new eyes—all discussing me.

I spent an entire day looking into bright lights, performing the standard tests of vision and answering questions. I went through many different eye exams with many different doctors. At the end of the day, I sat in on the seminar and lecture that this physician had come to deliver.

Doctor Croft had prepared a brief history highlighting my case. Listening to her give a synopsis of my descent into darkness along with all of the treatments, testing, and procedures that I had gone through was an incredibly humbling experience. The doctor that was giving the seminar had me stand, and I was honored by the attending physicians for my courage and attitude toward this life changing event. They thanked me for allowing them to be a part of it.

I always believed that Doctor Croft had my genuine interest at heart. She was always so helpful and caring. As Doctor Croft gave her findings, my knowledge of her level of caring and my undying respect for her could not have been higher.

It was because of this seminar that I ultimately was diagnosed with an energy failure disorder. The lecturing physician commented that he would send me to a rheumatologist who specializes in rare autoimmune disorders and diseases. The autoimmune specialist recognized the possibility of an energy failure disease and that led me to a specialist in Neuroimmunology.

He was highly educated on energy failure disorders and narrowed it down on our first meeting. He once again asked for more blood and a biopsy of muscle tissue in my leg. When I stopped at the lab for my 150th blood draw, they were confused by the orders. They had never seen these types of tests before and didn't know exactly how to prepare them.

They contacted the doctor, and he had to guide them through the setup, storage and transport of the different vials of blood. These tubes were sent off to labs in three different states because they were the only labs equipped to do the particular type of testing that he required. I should add, this specialized testing was not covered by insurance. The testing ranged from hundreds to thousands of dollars per test.

I had the biopsy in Feb of 2015, and you guessed it, on my wife's birthday. A small piece of muscle about the size of my pinky was removed from my left leg. This procedure left my leg numb. Between that and the three stroke-like episodes that I've had up to this point, I now have a permanent limp.

Throughout this arduous process, I was amazed and humbled by the entire group of doctors whom I associated with. I was blessed with a team of physicians who were at the top of their respective fields. They were all M.D.'s and had at least one, and most of them two, Ph.D.'s. One of the doctors who reviewed my case graduated medical school at age 17 and is in the Guinness Book of World Records for that accomplishment.

They all treated me like I was their main priority, although I knew they had many other patients. In their presence, even with all of my schooling, I felt like such an underachiever. Even in such perilous circumstances, I will always feel that it was a privilege and an honor to have associated with these magnificent people.

5

Blindsight

*"Right now everything looks so strange to me,
as if I don't belong here. It's me that's out of place.
And the worst thing is that I feel there's somewhere
I do belong, but I just can't find it."*

— L.J. Smith, The Awakening

People repeatedly tell me that they wish they could see through my eyes for one day, or ask me to describe what I see. Just as it was hard to explain how my body felt as it shut down, it's hard to explain what I see to people, when I don't understand it myself and haven't had the words to describe it. It is much like trying to describe what the color 7 tastes like.

I have given this much thought over the past two years and have come up with something that makes sense, in my mind anyway. To give others an idea, I have to give a better understanding of what's happening with my vision. I'll give you a brief explanation of the neuroscience behind it.

Most people do not realize that over a third of the brain is dedicated to vision. When you look at something, that's not necessarily what you see. Your brain has to discern the differences in the colors, shapes, distance, size and whether there is movement or not. All of those things come into your eyes as different photons of light and have to go to different portions of your brain. Each one of those portions determines all of those factors separately and then bring them together into one picture that you see—or that you believe you see.

Probably the most fascinating aspect of vision is your eyes have little to do with what you see. They are only the lens of the camera; they bring the light in, focus it on the receptors in the back of your eye, and then transfer that information to your brain. Your brain interprets that information and your mind creates the picture of what is in front of you. So *imagine* that you are looking at a black dog running across a bright green lawn in the middle of summer with fluffy white clouds floating by in a blue sky.

If there was a monitor on your brain during that exercise, the same areas of your brain would have lit up as would have if that were *actually* occurring in front of you. In other words, your brain does not know the difference between what you are visualizing in your mind and what you see through your eyes. According to your brain, both of them are vision. The most important thing is that you only see a tiny percentage of what you look at; the largest percentage is a construction in your brain.

Your hearing works in much the same way, and your brain doesn't know the difference between the two; it's just sensory stimulus coming in. There have been hundreds of experiments using other sensory input to create vision, even including the mouth. Studies have shown that one sensory input can be substituted for another. The blind have regained vision using both touch and electrical stimulus in the mouth.

The brain can also transfer the inputs and mix the senses without any external stimulus. Keep this in mind when we discuss my ability to see sounds in a later chapter.

We all have blind spots in our vision as well. The blind spot is where the optic disc or nerve bundle attaches to the back of your eye. There are no vision receptors in that area, therefore, no image detection. Each eye's blind spots are in different places. This allows one eye to compensate or help cover up the blind spot in the other eye. Our mind then includes those blank spots by accessing the information of the surroundings and filling it in with what it believes would match the rest of the picture.

To see this for yourself, try this test; hold your hands directly out in front of you at arm's length with your thumb and index finger in an 'L' shape, fingers pointing up. Touch your thumbs together, close your left eye and with your right eye, focus on your left finger. Your right finger will disappear. You may have to move your fingers out and in slightly until you find the exact spot of the blind spot, but it will be there.

When you find that blind spot, you'll notice it's not just a big white or dark spot; you see whatever is behind your finger as if you can see right through it to the wall behind them. This is because your brain, much like Photoshop on a computer, has a cut and paste function, your brain copied the background and that image filled in the missing spot. We do not see the world as a full picture like that from a camera. We only see a small portion; the rest is much faster for your brain to recall an image than try to reconstruct that image every single time you look at it.

This cut and paste function also works on a larger scale as well. The brain recognizes things that have been looked at multiple times, and much like a DVD, it replays that vision in your mind. It's a much faster process than discerning the photons of light each time. Because of this, we miss certain aspects of things that are going on around us as well. These have all been studied in great lengths by neuroscientists.

Change blindness is where our brain uses this cut and paste function to its fullest. Say I take a picture of a tree in a forest with flowers and moss and hundreds of other trees in the background. Then I make two copies of the same picture, only I change one of them by inserting a giant gorilla. If I flash those two pictures on a screen, say for a half a second each, even though there is a significant difference between those two pictures, your brain quickly assesses that it is the same picture and replays the first image. The majority of people will never pick up on that difference. Because the brain's ability to recall is faster than reassessing the entire picture; when it sees the second image, it automatically remembers the first image; therefore, you never see the large gorilla. Our mind creates visions for us to keep us from seeing things that we don't need to see and adding in the things that we cannot see.

This is all essential to explaining my vision, I swear.

I find the cruelest joke, however, is the *manipulation* of my sight. Many different disorders can affect people who have lost their sight. One of those is known as blindsight. Blindsight is where, after being sighted, an individual loses their vision and can guess the color or shape of objects in front of them at higher than average percentage. The key word here is *'GUESS'*. It's their belief they can see what's in front of them, even though their condition doesn't allow that.

As a blind person, this is incredibly frustrating because after I lost my eyesight, I believed at one point that it was getting better. I thought I could see more than what I could the day before. The clearest and easiest one for me to describe is in the bathroom. If you remember, before cell phones, we spent most of our time in the bathroom staring at the wall directly in front of us. Now we stare at our cell phones playing games. I believe it's most people's *'Social Media'* time.

On my bathroom wall, directly adjacent to the toilet, is an intricate design with hundreds of lines. Before losing my eyesight, I would sit and look at those designs and try to make patterns out of them. Or I would find objects—similar to what we do with clouds—where you locate the elephant or a top hat as they float by on a summer's day.

Not only would I try to find the designs or shapes within those patterns, but I would also see a labyrinth that I needed to find my way through. I would follow the patterns from one point to another just to occupy my time. About six months into my vision loss when most of my vision had gone, I went into the bathroom, sat down, and since the phone was now a blur, stared straight ahead at that wall when the most miraculous thing happened.

I could see the wall.

There they were, just as plain as the nose on my face, all of those designs. I could trace them just like I did so many times in the past. I could see all of the intricate little details and all of the little shapes and animals that I had seen so many times on that wall in the past. It was a miracle! I couldn't believe it! After all the testing and treatments, my vision just cleared up on its own.

I would close one eye and then the other just to see if the patterns changed. I do this quite frequently because my left and right eye have such a distinct vision pattern. I can determine if my vision has changed for better or worse. I close my right eye, and I can see the upper left-hand portion of the object. Then switching eyes, I can see the lower left-hand portion of it. It was always the same, never changing, until then. As I sat there staring at the wall in my bathroom, it changed—I could see.

Later that week was my appointment with my doctor, and I could not wait to explain that my vision was getting better. Throughout that day, I walked around and closed one eye and then the other, looking at all the different objects in my house. It was the same, all the walls, the television, even people. I walked outside, and I was so excited my vision was getting so much better. I knew that this was the turning point. I would again be able to see all those wonderful, beautiful things that I had missed for the past six months. I knew I would be waking up from this nightmare very soon.

At my appointment, I explained how much better I could see and how I was so excited! They were optimistic as well, and once again, put me through all of the visual tests that I have been through so many times before.

Track the dot of light.

Push the button every time the little white light appears in the dark space.

Stare at the flashing colored lights.

How many blinking red lights?

Lastly, the standard eye exam with the reading of the eye chart and the dreaded bright light eye exam. At the end of all of the testing, I was told that not only did my vision not get better, it was worse.

Wait, worse? How is it worse? What's going on?

I can tell you the things that are in my house; I can describe them to you. I can point them out and tell you where they are; it had to be getting better. Through all of that, I realized that my brain was just trying to compensate for what I could no longer see. I was seeing visions of things that I had looked at so many times before. My brain, like an old computer screen that had a picture displayed for too long, had that image burned into it. I was only recalling those images that I had seen so many times in the past.

The brain is miraculous, but it also has a cruel sense of humor.

Along with the blindsight, I also have hallucinations. It's confusing to people when I try to describe how a blind person can see, especially something that isn't even there. Damn, that's even confusing to me. Sure enough, daily I will jump and squint at whatever that was running across the floor, or the thing crawling down my arm, just like any sighted person seeing a mouse or a spider.

It's becoming more common, and I'm getting better at ignoring it, but sometimes the hallucinations still take me by surprise.

Plus, what if one day it *is* real? Chances are I won't see that. It's a disorder known as Charles Bonnet Syndrome. Research suggests that up to 60% of people who have lost their vision will experience some form of C.B.S.

Basically, when you lose your sight, your mind loses information from your eyes, so the brain sometimes fills the gaps by releasing imaginary pictures, patterns or even old images it has stored.

This phenomenon helps to describe how I move around and how I see. If you were to come to my house and watch me walk around, you wouldn't believe that I was blind. I walk around just as quickly and efficiently as anybody else in my home. I've lived here for almost two decades and in that time I have learned where everything sits, where the stairs are, how many there are, how many steps down the hallway, where the bathroom, bedrooms, living room, and dining room are. I have known all of this for 20 years.

As I walk through my house, my brain automatically generates those visions for me as if I can see. I know where everything is, and I can walk around freely. Very seldom do I trip, fall, or run into anything, unless something gets moved or left out. My brain compensates for my lack of vision by accessing the same visual cortex and recalling those images for me as I walk around.

Here's a simple experiment for you to try: This test is easy, and it gives the best representation of how and what I see.

Have a friend stand about three feet in front of you, while holding four different colored markers or highlighters in their hand. Make sure they know the particular order of colors, but do not reveal them to you. Stare directly at his nose and don't move your eyes. Have your friend raise the markers directly out to his side at arm's length and while you continue to stare at his nose, name the colors of the markers in the correct order.

More than likely you will know that there's something there, and you will probably be able to determine that there are colors. However, you will probably not be able to name the colors or the order of those colors in his hand. Now have him slowly bring his hands in closer to your central vision. Eventually, you will start to see one or two colors. But until his hand comes into your direct vision, you will not be able to name all of the colors.

I do not have any peripheral vision at all, so this experiment doesn't work for me. However, when I look directly at that handful of markers, it's the same as when your friend held them out to his side. I know that they are there, and I am aware that there are multiple colors, but as long as they are together in one bundle, I cannot discern the difference in the colors unless, of course, there happens to be fluorescent orange, which is one of the colors I am able to see. I can usually pick that color out of anything, but other colors all blend together. If you separate each one of those pens and allow me to look at them individually, I can get pretty close to the color. But as long as all the colors are together—I have no idea.

6

Speak Up

"Silence, I discover, is something you can actually hear."

— *Haruki Murakami*

After getting an informal diagnosis of an energy failure disorder, rather than a vision disorder, I no longer had appointments with Doctor Croft at the Moran. The focus turned to other aspects of the disease, specifically the energy failure parts. We were now tasked with figuring out the progression of the disease and the advanced stages I could look forward to.

As I said earlier, throughout my life I had always worried about losing my vision. I felt that I could lose any other body part or even my hearing, as long as I didn't lose my sight. I was even comforted by advancements in science and technology, as new and improved replacement limbs and other devices became available, because I believed that I wouldn't lose out on my way of life, as long as I could see.

As my hearing loss progresses, I've realized that, out of the two, I would rather lose my sight. After losing my vision, I can still get around and function. I can get past some of the things that my sight gave me by other means. For me, losing my hearing has become the most frustrating part of this disease.

I watched as both my father and my father-in-law dwindled into deafness. My dad has been deaf for years and has refused to learn sign language or any other means of communication, simply because he is too stubborn to try. I watch as his frustration and confusion in trying to communicate with people around him grows. How it aggravates him until he finally gives in and says, *"Okay"* and walks away, still not knowing what was said.

Imagine an 82 year old man who is five foot nothing, or how he tells it—four foot eighteen, (five-foot-six)—which I don't believe he's ever been in his life. He has grey-white hair that's seldom combed and has a mind of its own and weighs in at about 105 pounds soaking wet. He creates a space where the only person he talks to is himself, wandering in no apparent direction, throwing his hands in the air and muttering loudly and incoherently to himself, thinking nobody else can hear. That's my dad.

I feel so much frustration when I can't hear what's going on around me. When there is so much noise that I can't discern what's being said. When I first started losing my hearing, I was chosen to use a specific ear implant to see if it would help.

This implant is not like the cochlear implants that we've all heard so much about. Cochlear devices are surgically implanted into the area of your brain that receives the audio signal. These devices do not work for me because they attach to the auditory nerve that connects your ear to your brain. Just like my eyes, my ears are perfect. They hear everything that comes in, but the nerve doesn't transmit that signal to my brain.

Even though I was a candidate for this new implant, after it was placed into my ear I noticed that it amplified the surrounding noise, but not the particular sounds I needed to hear. It was mechanical and electronic and nothing sounded the same as I remembered. It was also painful at times. Once it was placed, there wasn't a way to control the tones that it picked up. It would amplify all the high pitched frequency noises that hurt at a reasonable volume.

Sounds like a fork dropped on a countertop or dog nails clicking against hardwood floors. The sound of metal against metal or placing a pan in a sink—those are the sounds that I picked up, the high-frequency, ear piercing sounds.

It was like having one of those air horns used at sporting events right up against the side of my head. Every few minutes it was set off, allowing that high pitched burst of sound to penetrate every cell of my body. Where it was implanted directly into my ear, it could only be removed by a doctor. So at times, my only options were to deal with the painfully loud noise or turn it off and hear nothing.

It had volume control, but there was great disparity between each step. Off was like an earplug, stopping all sound. This worked out great when I wanted to be alone with my thoughts. I must say, I started to understand how my father appreciated control over his own world and solitude. The next step was my normal hearing without an aide. From there, it increased by threes, ending with rock concert level. These were all pre-programmed and not adjustable.

I remember one day, I was at the bank talking to a teller. As we were conversing, he was typing on his computer. All I could hear were those keys clicking; I could not hear a word that he said. Under normal circumstances, I can hear most male voices, especially the lower, deeper tones. The clicking of those keys amplified by the implant was so overwhelming; I couldn't hear his voice at all.

Because this hearing aid was placed right next to my ear drum, it would amplify the waves that entered my ear before hitting the tympanic membrane. This is the way most hearing devices work. Even though it had the capability of glass shattering volume, there were times that I still could not hear. It was as if it would just cut out or stop working. Not like when I turned the device off, which was like the earplug. There was just no sound at all.

When I explained this to the doctor, she was confused. She had never heard of this problem with this device. She contacted the manufacturer who suggested that we try a new appliance. Their only thought was the device just happened to be faulty. Even with a new implant, there were many instances that my hearing would just shut off.

After the thirty day evaluation, I returned to my doctor, and we discussed all of the adverse effects; high pitched sounds and not being able to hear voices over the background. There was nothing they could do to change that. We also discussed the fact that I could not hear at certain points; as if the device turned itself off during the conversation. We considered the possibility that the hearing loss was due to nerve damage and not my ear function. This explained why it would intermittently shut off. Even though the device was helping out by amplifying the sounds coming into my ear, those sounds didn't make it to the processor in my brain. If the nerve is not transmitting, it doesn't matter how loud it is; I won't hear it.

This issue was something she had never dealt with before. After some further testing on the nerve transmission, she concluded that at times I would not be able to hear. Also, when the nerve depleted to the point that it could no longer transmit any sound, I would become completely deaf.

This was confirmed by my specialist as well. My disorder in most cases affects both the auditory and the optic nerve. It's as if the wires in a house have been cut. The power is still there; it just can't get to the light to turn it on. He told me that eventually there would be no way of amplifying the sound enough to get through the nerve. I would have to start learning to adjust to my hearing loss like I had my vision loss.

As I was learning to adapt to my hearing loss, a new side effect began to take a much greater role. I realized it wasn't just my hearing that would fade in and out. As I started losing certain words in the midst of a conversation, I also realized that sometimes I would fade in and out of reality.

It's very similar to a seizure in nature; I call them, *'time shifts.'* Like everything else with this disorder, it's so rare that I haven't experienced enough in my life to have the words to describe some of the feelings. I relate everything to comic books, and a parallel universe is the easiest way to describe it. Like I'm somewhere else, in some other time or realm and when I come back, it takes a minute before I realize where I am, what's going on and I have no control over my emotions.

One of the first times this occurred, I was with my mother and my wife. We were on our way home from an event and decided to go to my mother's favorite place to eat. It was late in the evening, and we were tired and exhausted, but we wanted a break from driving. I told my wife my order, she then walked me to a table where I sat down and waited for them to join me with the food.

It was easier than trying to walk through the line with my stick and holding onto someone's elbow as I also tried not to trip over those cattle trails they make with the black retractable nylon straps. As I was sitting there waiting, I began to feel *'off.'*

My wife and mom brought the food over and sat down, and we started to eat. I hadn't taken one or two bites when my mother said, *"Are you okay?"* Although I couldn't answer, I did hear her ask. It was as if I was in a trance where I could hear everything going on around me but I had no means of response.

My wife realized there was a problem and started asking, *"Shawn!...Shawn! What's wrong?"* I could hear the concern in her voice. It was as if I was in another room listening to a television conversation between the actors. After a few seconds, I shifted back and was able to reenter their reality. The only answer I had for all of their questions and concern was, *"I'm going to cry."*

So there we are, sitting in the restaurant with twenty strangers, and I'm bawling like a newborn baby. Tears running down my face and unable to control it or stop. The hardest part was I had no idea why. I had no reason to be crying. I wasn't sad, I wasn't angry, I wasn't upset, I was just crying. This went on for about five minutes before I could get my emotions back under control. Throughout the remainder of the night and the following day it remained the same; I would start crying for no apparent reason.

I've had to learn to manage and deal with this. My emotions are no longer mine. I feel like that puppet that I described earlier, where there's somebody else pulling the strings. I can be laughing and enjoying myself one second, then burst into tears for absolutely no reason. I'm like a pregnant woman who starts to cry just watching a television commercial. Of course I'm not pregnant, but I sure understand the emotional swings.

Along with the time shifts, I also have seizures. I have abnormal partial seizures, because nothing about me is normal. Most seizures affect the entire brain, but partial seizures only have an impact on a small area. There are two types of partial seizures; one is simple where you do not lose consciousness and can remember what happened during the seizure. Afterward, there is a feeling of anxiousness and fear. The second is complex. This type you usually lose consciousness and do not remember the event.

I have both of these. Because my partial seizures only have an effect on a part of the brain, the symptoms vary depending on which part of the brain is affected. My father always told me, *"You always have an arm out and a leg up,"* and this is now literally true. My limbs will just shoot out and shake for no reason. My head will start jerking and tilting to one side and although I know it is happening, there is nothing I can do about it.

By far, the most painful symptom for me to deal with is, *'Trigeminal Neuralgia.'* After my first stroke-like episode, the left side of my face from my ear to my jaw remained numb and tingly and it still affects me to this day. For no apparent reason and at random, I will get excruciating pain in the side of my face. It drops me right to my knees and at times stops me from breathing.

Imagine the worst migraine headache, the worst brain freeze, and the worst tooth ache that you've ever had in your life. Combine those and times that pain by 100 and that would be close to the amount of pain that shoots through the side of my face at random.

During these periods, I have absolutely no control. I can't speak, hear or move. Everything shuts down, except the pain. I have no muscle control, no way of communication. It's very hard for me to get people to understand that it isn't my choice not to communicate during the episode. I simply don't have the ability.

It took a long time for my wife to understand this, too. I would grab the side of my head and curl up into a little ball dropping to the floor.

"Are you ok? What's wrong? Why will you not answer me?"

My wife would get angry and frustrated because I didn't respond. I couldn't tell her what was going on, but in her mind, I was just ignoring her and refusing to answer.

After it would go away and I came back to awareness, she would yell at me in frustration. *"Why will you not talk to me? All you have to do is answer me!"* All I could ever say is, *"I can't."* After being told that this was one of the ancillary symptoms of my disease it was easier for my wife and people around me to understand that when this particular symptom occurs it shuts down any and all forms of communication.

As hard as it is, the only thing to do is wait. They last between 30 seconds and two minutes, and believe me, it is the longest time of my life. I feel like it will never end, then it goes away, and I can go back to whatever I was doing before the onset.

With all of this, every day is a new experience for me. I never know what is in store or what new development will show up.

However, through all of it, I have learned to embrace the day. If it's a good day, I am thankful for that day. If it's a bad day, I am also thankful. I know even on those bad days, when I am in pain or out of energy, I am alive.

Pain is just my body's way of letting me know I am still fighting. This is a war and I am determined to win. Pain only happens when you fight and the pain reminds me that I need to keep fighting.

Part 2
The Old Me

7

Skating On Milk

"You certainly didn't ask for them, and you can't trade them, but out of the billions of human beings on our planet, they're the ones who know you best. They're the ones who cherish you, and whom you should cherish in return— whether they're your biological family or otherwise."

— *Unknown*

I was raised in a relatively large family in northern Utah. I say relatively large because in Utah, six children is average. My mom always said that she wanted twelve children, but after having six, she decided that when we all got married, she would have her twelve. I was the only boy, and I was right in the middle with two older sisters and three younger. There is a struggle with being the middle child in any family, trying to figure out where you fit in. Wanting to do what the older kids do, but still wanting the luxuries of being younger. With me those issues were escalated, to say the least, by the fact that I was the only male child in the midst of an estrogen fiesta.

My mother was a stay at home mom or 'homemaker'. My father, who doesn't have a high school education, worked three jobs to provide for his family. Even working as hard as he did, my dad's highest yearly income when I was a child was approximately $12,000—the average was $35,000. My mom was very creative in finding ways to make the money stretch payday to payday, taking care of us through all of the ups and downs. I realized very soon, however, that I was to be the subject of ridicule during my elementary years.

Having only sisters made hand-me-downs a real nightmare. Nowadays, guys wearing girls pants is a fashion statement, but in the 1970's and early 80's, it was not. When other kids were going on summer vacations across the U.S. and receiving all the newest and greatest toys and games, I relied on my imagination to get by.

My mom and dad met in the summer of 1953 at a drug store and coffee shop where my maternal grandmother worked. She was only 15 and he was 19. My mom would go to help my grandmother, and my dad and his friends would come into the store to get a drink or a sandwich, then go out back and tell tall tales, trying to one-up each other's stories. She says now that she was too young and naive to be dating.

They went together for two years and on July 8th, 1955, they were married. The wedding was performed in my mother's parents' home. My mom told me that my grandparents had always wanted the wedding to take place there. After the ceremony, they had a small reception then moved into an equally small house to start their life together. But the honeymoon didn't last very long. They were only married for four short months when on November 5th, 1955, my father was drafted into the U.S. Army during the Korean conflict. He left for six weeks of basic training at Fort Ord, California and in December, was shipped to Korea.

He didn't talk much about the time he served in Korea, other than he spent two weeks on border patrol in the D.M.Z. (non-combat zone following the North and South Korean border), and the rest of the time in Incheon, South Korea—an area that was occupied by the U.S. Army during the conflict. Incheon Harbor was a shipping port for supplies, mail, and other necessities, and my father was part of the security forces that guarded those essentials. He was there for 21 months and returned home in September of 1957. He was stationed at Fort Carson Colorado to finish out his tour, then discharged on December 6th, 1957.

While my dad was in Korea, my mom's sister and her husband were stationed in Texas. When her sister delivered her first son, my mom traveled to Texas to help out. This is one of my mom's favorite memories and as she likes to tell it, when she met Elvis. Well—sort of.

Elvis was stationed at the same base as her brother-in-law. While she was there visiting and helping her sister, she saw Elvis, in his uniform, drive by in his pink Cadillac. That's it, the whole story. Elvis just drove by. Like many women of her time, my mom has an unreasonable love for Elvis. To this day, she has an entire room in her house dedicated to Elvis—pictures, posters, statues, and albums. You name it, if it has anything to do with Elvis, she has it and it's displayed proudly in a room that no one is allowed to enter. Not only because it's priceless to her, and she doesn't want anything broken, but there's no room to move around. It's very organized, but full.

During their stay in Colorado, they rented a small studio apartment, and my dad would travel back and forth to the base while my mom stayed at home. My father was paid by the US Army $111 per month, the rent on the studio apartment was $33 a month. Since my mom was home all day while my dad was on base, they decided to rent a television so she would have some form of entertainment. The rent on the TV was $3 per month; gas was less than a quarter per gallon. After bills had been paid and the fridge and pantry were re-stocked, there wasn't much money left, which was a great learning experience and why she was always able to make the money stretch later in life.

When dad returned from Korea, they were excited to begin their family, and for the next six years, they tried to fulfill that dream. My father was diagnosed with a low sperm count. They spent countless hours and a lot of money attempting to solve this issue. My dad received several different treatments for both low testosterone and pituitary issues, which stimulate sperm production and restore fertility. In the spring of 1962, my mom saw an article in the newspaper advertising adoption, and they made an appointment with Children's Adoption Society in Ogden, Utah to start the process.

This was no small feat. They had to go to the center once a month to evaluate employment, marriage stability, extended family, and so on. In April 1963, my oldest sister was born, and on May 5th, she was delivered into my parent's arms. She had a dirty face and was crying, but they didn't care, she was all theirs and they would take her and bathe her and love her just as their own.

On the way home they heard the name Brenda on the radio, and she had a name. They had to wait for a year to legally adopt her, and one year later almost to the day, they stood in front of a judge in an old city courthouse and made everything official.

At the same time they were making Brenda's adoption legal, they returned to the Children's Adoption Society again. The year-long process of background checks and jumping through legal hoops started all over, until they could receive a child. November 1965 my second sister was born, and three days later, she was welcomed into the family. My parents had a hard time naming her and for six weeks she was just known as *'baby girl.'* One day, someone commented how she was a little jewel—the name Julie stuck. Once again, a year later, they were back at the Ogden courthouse making Julie's adoption legal.

Even though both of my older sisters were adopted, we never believed them to be anything other than sisters; just as much family as biological siblings. We didn't give it a second thought. My sisters always said that this was their family and it didn't matter who gave birth to them.

My mom likes to tell the story of how I was conceived. No, I'm not turning this into a graphic novel or pornographic escapade, but I find it quite amusing and feel it's worth telling. In late September 1967, my parents, sisters and my mother's parents took a trip to

Yellowstone National Park. They rented and shared a cabin. My sisters were only four and two respectively. Apparently my father started getting frisky, and mom was trying to stay quiet and not wake her parents. Even though they were all in the same room, he would not be deterred. The next morning she was so embarrassed that she wouldn't even look her parents in the eye.

My grandparents never acted as if they knew anything, so she continued the day as normal. Mom said the reason she got pregnant was because she was so petrified. My sister Julie became ill while they were in Yellowstone, requiring the need of a doctor, and they returned home early. Julie ended up needing her tonsils removed, and when my mom kept getting sick trying to take care of her, she realized she was pregnant.

June, 1968, after eleven years of trying and seeing doctor after doctor for help, I was brought into this world. I was the first biological child, and I put my mother through 26 hours of labor. Even then I was stubborn and failed to recognize there's an easier way of doing things.

I was born with a literal point on my head as well as something that was going to define who I was and how I would live my life, though no one knew it was there—one small genetic marker, one tiny mutation. It was to change my life 35 years later. There were all kinds of minor abnormalities throughout my life, but it wasn't until I was 40 years old that I realized all of those tiny little defects added up to the big one that I was going to have to live with.

When I was four years old, I had been suffering from tonsillitis and was admitted to the hospital, where my tonsils were removed. Back then, people were admitted to the hospital for several days after even the smallest surgeries. My mom would come up to the hospital to sit with me because I was whining a lot; apparently I was a cry baby. She was rescued from my incessant crying and complaining when she went into labor with my younger sister. She later told me she went into labor because the women delivering were crying less than I was, so it would be a relief. November, 1972 my third sister was born.

The doctor believed my mom was pregnant with twins because there was a heartbeat echo that sounded like two heartbeats and there weren't ultrasounds back then. When Luci was born, mom was slightly disappointed because she always wanted twins.

My fourth sister was born March, 1975. One week before her birth, my mom started having pains and went to the hospital. The doctor said it was too early, sent her home and put her on bed rest. The pains continued and Mom returned to the hospital. When Sherry was born, she was blue from lack of oxygen; the umbilical cord was wrapped around her neck twice.

The doctor said she may have died if she had not delivered when she did. Mom initially didn't get to hold Sherry and Dad didn't even get to see her as they rushed her off to the Neonatal Intensive Care Unit. They placed her in an oxygen rich incubator where she remained for three days, and my parents could only see her through the window of the unit and the glass of the incubator.

My fifth and final sister was born in March 1977, on the first day of Spring. Because of this, my dad was adamant about naming her Spring. However, his mother asked if they would name her after my dad's middle name, which is Rahn, pronounced *"Ron."* She was named Rhonda Spring. Grandma wanted it spelled like my father's—Rahnda—but my mother thought there would be too much confusion and spelled it the traditional way.

When we were young, my sisters and I were very close; we did everything together from camping to building snowmen in the yard to even playing dolls. My sisters would be playing house with their baby dolls, and I wanted to play, too. But I was left out, because I was a boy. They wouldn't let me near any of their precious dolls, so my parents decided I needed one of my own to stop the fighting.

What did they get me? Not a Ken or even a G.I. Joe—which back in the day was just one man and not a whole team like it is now. No, the doll I got was a Raggedy Andy, which looked like an Amish version of Ronald McDonald with his red curly hair, overalls, and painted on scarecrow face. None of them wanted to play with it because it was a boy doll, but since there was a need for a dad in their make-believe home, TA-DA, I got to be the only unwanted doll in the room. Of course, I was always told what to do and what to say, and try as I would, none of my input was ever accepted.

I got even with them, though. Whenever my parents would leave, my two older sisters were charged with babysitting. This led to a lot of fighting between us because I was defiant as a mule and just as stubborn. Some of our fights could be quite lengthy and even brutal. My sister Julie will tell you how, in one of the more epic battles, I punched her so hard that she couldn't breathe. To this day, I have a hard time with face creams, lotions and even some perfumes because once, they held me down and poured baby powder all over my face. We still loved and cared for each other, but we were typical siblings fighting for our place in the family.

Of course, we didn't always fight. There were many nights that we had to create our own fun and excitement, and this is where I excelled. I would often come up with some scheme including a yet undiscovered game or pastime. There is one that I am particularly proud of. We had roller skates. Not the inline or even the four wheel skates that are popular today. These were simple hunks of metal that were fastened together with a center screw, allowing them to be adjusted longer or shorter depending on the size of your foot.

Attached to that were four steel wheels that revolved around a steel rod which was welded to the center frame. If you splurged and spent the extra two dollars, you could have ball bearings, but we didn't have that kind of money.

There were leather straps that we'd buckle over our shoes and around our ankles. Then we'd turn the special key that tightened them down onto our foot and, Voila! We could skate almost as fast as we could walk and with only twice the effort.

Pretty sure it was winter, and it was dark, so we couldn't skate outside. That's when I had the brilliant idea to roller skate in the house. Now my older sisters weren't going to allow that to happen. Those skates would only tear up the carpet and ruin the floor in the kitchen, and they were not about to be the sisters who allowed me to tear up the house.

I decided that there had to be a way. I ditched the skates and put on a pair of socks and started sliding across the kitchen floor. Our kitchen wasn't very long, so I would get just a couple of steps in, then slide. But I was only sliding a foot or two and it was more dragging than sliding.

My sisters thought this was a great idea and joined in, each of us trying to out-do the other on distance. This is where the actual fun began. I decided that the floor was too dry, and if it were wet, we would have less traction and thereby, slide faster and farther. Hey, even at 10, my head wasn't just a hat rack. My sisters agreed with my theory, but decided we needed more room to get a better start. So the three of us moved the kitchen table and chairs into the living room and started the process of building a skating rink, right in our home. After careful deliberation, it was decided that water wasn't going to give us a slippery enough surface, so I suggested that we use milk.

Back then my parent's floor was linoleum. A lot like today's vinyl, but much more durable. Linoleum is made with linseed oil which, when liquid is added, well—let's just say it was better than using the roller skates. My sisters and I were sliding from one end of the kitchen to the other as fast as we could, feeling like rockets flying out of the earth's gravity. The only thing stopping us was the wall, and at times, rather abruptly.

We were having the time of our lives, and all it took were some socks and two gallons of milk. We were covered, along with the walls, cupboards, carpet; even the dog, because she was trying to lick up our newly found playground. When my parents came home, we were excited to show them how much fun we were having! We just knew that they would want to run right to their room and put on some socks and join in the fun. Surprisingly, our hopes of further play were quickly, and quite literally, mopped up.

8

I Am Iron Man

"But I remember one thing: it wasn't me that started acting deaf, it was people that first started acting like I was too dumb to hear or see or say anything at all."

— Ken Kesey, One Flew Over the Cuckoo's Nest

When I was a child, I was considered to be the obnoxious type. I was constantly moving and doing something. My brain was always moving from one topic to another, I had a hard time focusing and I was extremely hyperactive. That was the term used back then, *'Hyperactive!'* There wasn't A.D.D. or the more popular A.D.H.D. Back then it was a lack of discipline or lack of education that caused such behaviors. Well, I can assure you there was no lack of discipline in my home growing up, and my education, although my teachers probably wouldn't agree, was typical.

Countless times, an obscure question would plague a friend or family member, or the occasional game night question and answer hour, where I could, in the words of my family, pull the correct answer out of a particular body part not usually used to store information.

SHAWN PAULSEN

How did I do this? Where did the information come from?

I was labeled as having a low I.Q. and unteachable by the education system. I was treated as inferior by family members because of this disorder. Yet, somewhere and somehow this information was stored in some part of my brain. To this day, my friends call me the 'Master of D.U.I.'—*Doctrine of Useless Information*. For whatever reason, I can retain strange and useless facts that I have learned, all the while being accused of not paying attention.

There were many children just like me, all lumped into a pile called, *'unteachable and out of control'*, and most of us suffering from self-esteem issues. Of course, those beliefs have changed. There have been numerous studies conducted on the effects of A.D.D. and A.D.H.D. and how to better help these disorders. They are now referred to as learning disabilities, and the idea of I.Q. and education and treatment of these children has significantly changed.

In the 1950 and 60's, children born with physical and mental disabilities were doomed to life in an institution. Doctors and other health care professionals were at a loss as to what to do with these children. They were locked away and their parents told to forget them and just move on with their lives, but these beliefs no longer hold true. We have come to learn that most of these children are brilliant; capable of learning, speaking, and other great feats that weren't believed before.

I had the great opportunity of teaching in a classroom of children labeled handicapped. The classroom held children between five and twelve years, with a myriad of both physical and mental disabilities. In the three years I spent in that room full of beautiful little angels, I learned more about my life and the beliefs that I had regarding disabilities than I ever thought possible.

The tenacity and determination that these children possessed went beyond anything I had ever seen in my life. They were brilliant and talented young people, and they deserved to have every opportunity afforded to them. Yet inside the same school that they attended were bigotries and assumptions about their abilities. Every single day, those children taught me something new about myself, my abilities and my disabilities.

Although I don't agree with all of today's interventions, I have to wonder where I would be now if some of these ideas had been used with me, all those many years ago? Would I have gone to school and continued my education through to my doctorate? Would I have been able to succeed in my two professional careers? Would I be writing this book?

When I was a child, I would play *'Cops and Robbers'* or *'Cowboys and Indians'*, just as most children do. However, I would also play pretend games in my head that absolutely *cannot* be real. But, in my world, I honestly believed *could* be real, if I just believed in them hard enough.

For example, I would spend hour upon hour in make-believe worlds, where I could fly or lasers would shoot out of my hands. I took *'Neverlands'* and *'Avatars'* to the most extreme, believing they were real. In my mind, they existed.

I had visions of levitation and telekinesis. I could change the channels on the television with my mind because I *believed* it could be true. The strange thing about this is, it proved very useful in my career as a standup comic and therapist.

Think about the nearly endless list of comic book heroes—Spiderman, Superman, X-Men. They all had one thing in common with me. They were all nerds, left out, ridiculed or otherwise outcast in some way. But in their minds, they developed a way to overcome all of that and be the hero, the envy of the common man and the fear of the oppressors of the world. Comic books and heroes are the result of my kind of childhood.

Video games are another example. In the video gamer's world, they are the hero. The scene is acted out on the screen in front of him or her for the whole world to see and understand. This escape from reality claims more and more people, not just those with A.D.H.D. We are all looking for something in life to believe in, or that proves who we are and why we are here. We can find the self-esteem we all search for and need to survive, and the acceptance of others, even if the *'others'* are from the make-believe world we share.

I loved and still love comic books, science fiction and anything that enables people to overcome adversity and become stronger or smarter. Growing up, it was my escape from my father or the neighborhood bullies. As a young man, my hero was Ironman. He was an everyday guy—well, if being uber smart and a billionaire is everyday—who made his superpowers via a metal suit. Of course, having rockets and lasers were kind of cool, too.

If I just tried hard enough, I thought, it would come true for me as well. All I had to do was believe, and those energy beams would shoot right out of my hands just like Ironman. I could protect myself from all the bad people in my life and then fly off with my rocket boots and go where I could do some good in the world. I loved other heroes as well, but Ironman was my guy.

I learned to tell stories because of my childhood. I felt inferior because of my hyperactivity and family issues, and I wanted desperately to be accepted and fit in. All I wanted was to be loved and thought of as someone that people wanted to be around, but this wasn't the case. For most of my life, hyperbole has been a means of communication. My father was quite a storyteller; he always had an active imagination, and everything was always larger and greater than it really was.

This flawed character trait that my father was so good at wielding, I learned to use in my life. Most of the time it didn't create problems and no one got hurt by the grandiose nature of my stories. I would often exaggerate. Size, amounts, anything that I felt would make me feel like someone other people would want to be around. The fish I caught were always twice the size and twice the number. The shots I made were always too easy, or my abilities on a bicycle or a skateboard were incredible. I believed that the bigger the story, the more fascinating I could make myself, and people would want to be around me more. Unfortunately, it didn't work like I thought. The more I exaggerated, the more people saw through me. Yet I continued. It's nothing I'm proud of now, but it is part of my life and something that I have worked to overcome.

We are all guilty of exaggerating to make a point or as a way of understanding a particular situation from time to time, but for me, it was normal conversation.

I never had any intentions of malice, nor was it my intent to mislead anybody or to create a false identity for monetary reasons. It was merely something that I learned when I was very young, and it was tough for me to stop. As I grew into adulthood, it followed me. I was self-deprecating and had a lack of self-esteem. For some reason, in the back of my mind, I was looking for some form of greatness.

As I traveled the countryside as an adult from comedy club to comedy club, state to state, I would dream up identities for myself. I would change where I came from. I would have complete backgrounds and history for myself for each of the locations. For me, it was a fun game and at the same time, a way of trying to gain acceptance. I've portrayed myself as being an orphan, a world traveler and everything in between. Some of these identities became part of my everyday life.

I realize now it was a means of self-preservation, wanting to be something that I wasn't, just like those comic book characters wanted to be something better. I was always trying to prove that I was something, but in reality, I made myself into nothing. I have since learned to overcome this huge stumbling block of mine. I've accomplished so much in my life to be proud of. At the time I was going through this, I never understood why. However, I finally realized I was looking for the acceptance of my father.

I no longer need to make up stories or embellish to prove who I am or what I'm worth. A made-up life can't even compare. I wish I would have learned this lesson earlier. I could have had a much better relationship with friends and loved ones. I am now aware, late in this life, that who I am is enough, and it's okay for me to be me. I don't have to prove anything to anyone, except myself. I no longer need to run and hide within my own mind so that someone will like me…including me.

The biggest lie I lived can be said in a single statement, *"I don't care what anybody else thinks."* I lived my life that way; convinced other people that I didn't care what they or anyone thought, and in reality, that was a painful thing for me to do. I **"DO"** care what everybody else thinks. I want to be accepted; I want to be loved; I want to be looked up to and be a person that other people want to emulate.

I spent many hours in therapy trying to understand some of the mind-boggling reasons for my actions. I knew what I was doing, but I was afraid of who I was. I was petrified that somebody would find out what I was like; how scared, lonely and depressed I was.

All of those stories, all of those false lives, were all built just like those comic books. I was the underdog, the one left behind, and all I wanted was to save the world.

I had no idea who I was! And I wanted no one to ever know the full story of my life—until now.

9

Dr. Jekyll and Mr. Hyde

"At what point does a man turn into a monster? I don't believe that it's when he does horrible things, but when he accepts that he's able to do them, and that he does them well."

— *John Greenleaf Whittier*

My father was a disciplinarian, and he believed that his way was the only way. In my house, my father set the rules and firmly established the idea that his way was forged in time, blood, sweat, and tears, and there wasn't any other possible alternative. It was the only way he knew. Therefore, it was true. Being the only boy, I was held responsible for most of the problems and things that went wrong in the home.

This is not to say that I wasn't the one who instigated some of the situations that caused me great grief. However, the punishment became harsher and more abusive for me. My father believed that abuse was the way to prove that he was the boss.

When my father returned from Korea, Mom told me he wasn't the same man. He was suffering from what would now be diagnosed as P.T.S.D. Once again, in the late 1950's, that wasn't something that was discussed, let alone diagnosed. The nightmares and paranoia were very prominent for many years after he returned home.

Mom told us stories of how he would wake up in the middle of the night screaming and swinging his fists, and at times throwing things. Other times he would toss and turn with nightmares, breaking things in their headboard.

I pause here for just a moment to talk about my father. I do not wish to portray him as a tyrant, or being abusive to the extent of needing to be removed from the home. However, if I portrayed him in any other light, it would be a lie. My father was institutionalized several times.

He had his way of doing things and, in his mind, there was no other way. For my father, I was a great embarrassment as a child. I always did things wrong, I was always in his way and everything was my fault. Some of you reading this may become very upset with how harshly he treated me. I have repeatedly been asked why they let him back into the home, or why Mom never left him? In the 1970's, child protective services wasn't what it is today. In many cases, people just turned their heads to the punishment administered to both children and women.

Mom was not only extremely faithful, but she felt she didn't have any other means of survival. The mental abuse kept her believing that she could never find anyone else, and she was dedicated to her children, so she stuck it out.

I also admit that no one in my family knew what my father did to me. I was silent until I suffered my first stroke-like episode. That's when many of the childhood memories came flooding back, and I couldn't be silent any longer. My sisters and mom knew that he was hard on me, but they didn't see the abuse, and, to be honest, they probably felt I deserved it. Recently I have come to learn more about him and have forgiven him for a lot of his actions.

When I was about ten years old, we were getting ready to go on a camping trip. We had a utility trailer that we would occasionally use to gather trash for the dump. We wanted to use it for this trip, but it needed to be emptied. My father and I took it to the local landfill and emptied it. On the way home our trailer came off the hitch.

DR. JEKYLL AND MR. HYDE

I don't remember exactly how, whether it wasn't locked down or if the hitch broke—I guess it doesn't matter, it just came unhitched. It started dragging down the road causing the vehicle to swerve out of control and digging a gouge in the roadway with the tongue. This upset my father a great deal, as you would expect. However, what you wouldn't expect is why.

My father wasn't angry because the trailer came loose, or the fact that it was damaged and we could no longer use it for the trip, or even at the thought of the cost of fixing it. It was that he believed I should have known that it had come loose and alerted him before it came off. The fact that I was sitting in the front seat of the truck right alongside him and looking out the front windshield just as he was never crossed his mind.

All he could see was that it was my responsibility to somehow use my *'spidey-sense'* to see into the future and know that it was going to happen. Then use my *'Flash'* abilities to move back there with lightning speed and with the strength of *'The Incredible Hulk'* keep it from happening. In my father's eyes, this was my fault entirely.

My father was determined to get the trailer home under any circumstances. He knew that we needed it to go on the trip and also that if a law enforcement officer found it on the side of the road it could be towed and, even worse, tracked back to him and he'd be fined for the road damage. My father's solution to this was simple; he removed the spare tire from underneath the truck and placed it into the bed. He then took the trailer tongue and raised it just below the tailgate so that the safety chains of the trailer could be wrapped around the spare tire to hold it in place.

The tongue of the trailer was now free-floating behind the truck attached to a tire that was resting in the bed of the pickup, by the safety chains. My father, realizing that the tire would not be substantial enough to hold the trailer in place, added a 75 pound ten-year-old boy to the rear of the pickup truck. I believe his initial thought was that I was to use that imagined *'Hulk-like'* strength to hold the tire in place while he drove home.

This was not an incredibly heavy trailer; however for a boy of 10, it may as well have been Thor's hammer.

After only a few feet of driving, my father realized I was not capable of holding onto the tire and the weight of the trailer, as the tire slipped from my arms and the trailer and tire both careened off the roadway once again. This made my father even angrier because I should have been strong enough to hold it. He informed me that when he was my age, he would have been able to pick up the trailer and carry it home.

Once again, he set up his towing package in the way he did before, however, this time, to ensure that we would make it back, he found a second set of chains and fastened me to the spare tire that the trailer was attached to. Before we started down the road the second time his only statement to me was, *"You better hope it doesn't come out."*

I quite literally held on for dear life. I knew that if the trailer pulled the tire out of the back of the pickup truck, I would be going with it and then I would get drug down the roadway as the spare tire did just moments ago. My muscles ached and burned as the tire dug into the insides of my legs and arms.

My grip was all I had to hold it in place. The skin was rubbed away from the inside of my arms as the tire would jerk back and forth. This only went on for a short distance when my father realized that other cars were passing by and were staring at this 10 year old boy in the back of his pickup, chained to a trailer.

My father pulled over to the side of the road, disconnected the trailer and me, and we drove home. The entire trip back I was lectured on how this was entirely my fault, and if I had been able to hold on to that trailer, we would have been home by now. I also had a firm understanding that I was to tell nobody what had just happened.

I don't believe this was because he felt he would get in trouble for what he did. I think he was embarrassed by my failure once again. And in case you are wondering what happened to the trailer,

DR. JEKYLL AND MR. HYDE

my father left it on the side of the road and picked it up after our camping trip.

My father was extremely competitive, and he made it a point to let me know on every occasion possible. One evening I was at my cousin's home who lives right next door to my parents. It was late and my father had come over to retrieve me for the night.

My aunt had beautiful rose gardens in front of her home which she meticulously kept. There was also a cluster of roses between our house and my cousin's house forming a hedge-like fence. As we exited my cousin's home, I immediately started running towards my house knowing that the sooner I could get there, get ready for bed, and get to sleep, the less likely that night's beating would occur.

My father, not to be outdone, ran behind me as if it were a race to get home. As I ran across my cousin's front yard, my father closed the distance between us, shoving me in the back and into the hedge of roses. The thorns and limbs of the rose bushes dug into my body covering me with cuts and scratches.

As I screamed in pain, my father reached into the roses, grabbed my shirt and staring at me with a smile on his face, yanked me back out of the roses without trying to remove any of the limbs first. Again, my body was cut, scratched and punctured. I was bleeding and had rose thorns still embedded in me as he carried me into the house.

With a very concerned look on his face, he told my mom how I was not paying attention and ran right through the middle of those roses. I never corrected him or tried to explain what happened. I only said it was dark, and I didn't see them.

I have never really been into traditional sports like baseball, football, and soccer. However, I did play all of them at some point in my childhood. As much as my father was never there for me, my mom always was. She attended every game, practice and team meeting; she supported me in every way.

There was the rare occasion that my father would show up to one of the games and these times were both nerve-racking and exciting for me. As much as I always wanted my father there, I knew if I didn't play well he would be there to rub it in and make it worse for me. It was either *"You lost the game and let down your entire team!"*, or *"They only won because the coach was smart enough not to play you."* It was never, *"Great job, son."*

When I was about 12 years old, I was playing little league baseball. There was an older boy in the park, and he and I didn't get along. He threw me to the ground while my team was at bat and began the typical torture; knuckling my sternum and spitting on my forehead. When our team returned to the field, I tried and tried to get out from under the older boy who had my shoulders pinned down with his knees, but to no avail.

My father saw what was happening and came to my rescue, or so I thought. While he did get the boy off of me and got me to the field, he lectured me the entire time about how I was an embarrassment to him, and how I let the team down again. No matter how I tried to argue that I was trying, and it wasn't my fault, my father grew angrier with me.

After the game, I assumed it was over and forgotten, but you know what they say about assuming. I should have known that is not how my father saw it. When we got home, he promptly lead me out to the backyard and as he saw it, taught me how to fight so I wouldn't embarrass him again. His way of teaching me was punching me in the face and stomach. As I lay on the ground trying to see and catch my breath, he walked away saying, *"Maybe that will teach you something."*

My father also took out his frustration on inanimate objects, in a very backward and destructive way. My parents were remodeling their basement after all of us had moved out and on with our lives. He had put up sheetrock and wood, painted and carpeted, and had created a very comfortable family room. They got new furniture and Dad wanted the old furniture out. It was at this time I received one of the many calls I get from my mother since I've become an adult and am better able to deal with my father. It went something like this:

ME: *"Hi mom."*
MOM: *"Shawn, you need to get over here right now! Dad is tearing down my wall!"*
ME: *"What?"*
MOM: *"Dad is trying to move the old couch out of the new family room, and it won't go through the door, so he is tearing out the wall to get it through!"*
ME: *"I'll be right there."*

This isn't the first time that I had to go and save the house or car or multiple other objects that fell prey to my father's *'Fuck It!'* attitude. When I arrived, I found my father taking a sledgehammer to the brand new wall that he had just finished. All because the couch was stuck. I immediately stopped the carnage and asked very calmly…okay, more like…

"DAD! WHAT IN THE HELL ARE YOU DOING!?" To which the answer that I have heard all too many times…

"THIS DAMN THING IS STUCK, AND THERE IS NO OTHER WAY TO GET IT OUT!"

As I said, my father had one way of doing things, and it was correct no matter what. So after wrestling the hammer out of his grasp, I calmly asked if he had tried to remove the legs. By the look on his face, I knew the thought of removing the legs never crossed his mind—until now.

Being that his way is always right and that he cannot be at fault, he answered by saying, *"These legs are part of the frame, and they won't come off!"* He stated this with certainty and authority so as to take all doubt away, convincing me that we shouldn't even try to take them off, for fear of the dreaded wrath of Dad and *"I told you so, you don't ever listen!"*

It was at this point that I took it upon myself to test his theory. As I reached for the leg to give it a twist, I heard, very sternly, *"I told you I have already tried that, and they won't come off!"* But this time in a more, *'Don't you dare prove me wrong,'* tone that I was *SO* afraid of as a child. It is amazing to me, in retrospect, how it wasn't necessarily the things that my father said to me that made me believe, fear, or even at times admire him. It was his *tone* which influenced me so much.

Being an adult and having the ability to argue intelligently with my father, I did the impossible. I reached out and unscrewed the couch legs. I had complete faith as to the answer that my father would give to this astounding feat, thus I was not disappointed when I heard, *"Well, I tried that and they wouldn't come off for me!"*

I have found that lecturing my father is like attempting to convince a plant that it can grow multiple colored flowers when all it has ever done is grow single color flora. But still, it makes me feel better.

ME: *"Dad, what were you thinking?"*
DAD: *"There wasn't any other way; I couldn't get the legs off."*
ME: *"This couch is going to the landfill right?"*
DAD: *"Yes, it's 40 years old, and it is completely broken."*
ME: *"Then wouldn't it have been more logical to cut the old and useless couch in half and remove the halves rather than destroying the new wall that you now have to finish again?"*
DAD: SILENCE......

This was typical of my father. I watched as hammers, saws, and other tools of destruction were used. I watched as parts and pieces of tables, cars and a multitude of objects were destroyed because he couldn't control his anger. As a child, it meant that my toys and other valuables would get destroyed in fits of rage if left out or not taken care of as he wanted.

I was forced to watch as he dismantled my bicycle. I say dismantled but a better description would be that he threw it down on the driveway, took a hammer to what didn't break off, then tossed it in the trash. All because I was riding it in the roadway, and it caused a car to have to slow down and, in his words, *"You weren't paying attention and almost got killed!"* Therefore I wasn't responsible enough to have a bike.

DR. JEKYLL AND MR. HYDE

Clearly, my father and I didn't have a very positive relationship as I was growing up. As I got older, it grew worse, and we drifted further apart. The only thing I could see was this evil tyrant who caused my life to be hell. I now believe that everything happens to us so that we can learn from the experience and take something positive from it. But at that time, I couldn't find any good in him or those experiences. There was a point where my father could have died, and I wouldn't have attended his funeral.

He has since been diagnosed with Paranoid Schizophrenia and Dementia. These diagnoses have helped me sort out the issues that my father and I had. I learned that I needed to find the good in my father and to work with the situation at hand. Through my mental unfolding, I was able to look at my life and separate my father into two personalities. I chose Dr. Jekyll and Mr. Hyde.

Through this analogy, I could put all of the negative things that I experienced with my father in one basket and label it Mr. Hyde. By doing this, I could better see the good qualities and fun activities that we had growing up, which I put in a basket and labeled Dr. Jekyll. I was able to release my guilt over the Mr. Hyde experiences and give the responsibility back to my father for his actions. They were not my fault.

They also weren't entirely his fault, based on his diagnosis. Finally, I could see that Dr. Jekyll was my dad, and Mr. Hyde was the mental disorders. By allowing my beliefs to change and getting some release from the guilt that I felt, I was able to have the relationship with my dad that I longed for as a child. I now have tons of good memories, and I am a much better person because of it.

My dad was the dad my friends loved and wanted to be around. He was the dad who played with the neighborhood kids. A grown man playing cops and robbers, and telling us stories and anecdotes that all the children loved. There were also camping trips, hunting and fishing, nights of bowling, and family craft nights. There are many great times that I now remember and cherish because of the changes I made in my own life.

10
Mom Said I Would Never See 13

"I never look back darling; it distracts from the now."
— Edna Mode, The Incredibles

When I was younger, I was always running around the neighborhoods, riding my bike, and climbing trees. I even rode my bicycle out of a tree. Yes, I said out of a *TREE*. Well, actually it was a tree house—a really awesome tree house. My friends and I spent an entire summer collecting wood—okay, stealing wood—from the subdivisions that were building up around us. We chose a friends backyard to build this treehouse because he had a really, really tall old tree.

This was no ordinary tall tree. This was a monster tree, with massive arms for limbs and a base big enough to play hide and seek behind with Big Foot. For a 12 year old boy, this was huge! We had enough room for all five of us, a television and gaming system, (I say system but in reality, it was the first Pong and a 12" black and white television, so system is probably pushing it a bit) a couch, and chairs, and even with all this, we could still move around.

We constructed walls and built windows. Picture the movie 'Sandlot' and the scene in the treehouse where they are overlooking

MOM SAID I WOULD NEVER SEE 13

the fenced yard with the enormous dog. Now you have an idea of what our house looked like, with one exception—we had a garage.

Yes, we built a garage for our bicycles. You can't just leave those things laying around. We had a pulley system where one of us would climb halfway up the tree, another of us would be in our *'garage'* and the rest of us were on the ground where we would tie a rope to the bike in a way that would keep the bike as level as possible. The job of the person halfway up was to guide the bike through the limbs of the tree to the garage. The kid in the garage would then untie the bike and send the rope back to the ground, where the process started all over again. At the end of the day, we went in reverse and would lower the bikes to the ground, then make our way home.

We spent from sun-up to sun-down (and sometimes the entire night), all summer in that treehouse. One day, while in the midst of this tedious bicycle routine, we thought there had to be an easier way to do this. A ramp was started but quickly abandoned as we realized that the ramp would have to go into the street to get the angle right, and we didn't have enough material to support it. I know this because we tried to use the ramp and fell right through. Another thought was to just throw the bikes out of the tree. We came up with several other ideas, but it came down to a 12-year-old boy's imagination and a dare.

Of course, I was the 12-year-old boy and I had one hell of an imagination. In my mind, if we got on our bikes in the garage and started peddling and rode the bike out of the tree, we would land on the ground, still peddling, and just keep on going. I saw nothing wrong with this idea because I witnessed it every Saturday morning on cartoons. It was perfect.

I would ride out of the garage and fall gracefully to the ground. Then I would go off into the sunset with the admiration of all my friends. After some laughter and the dare I mentioned, I decided that it would be better to get a running start off the slanted roof of the treehouse.

You need to realize that even though this was a large tree house, the roof was still only slightly longer than my bike. So the running start was more like a step. I made one full pedal, and suddenly the bike and I were on our way to the ground. Now, take a moment to recall the old Looney Tunes cartoons, where a character would be walking or riding at the end of a building and instead of continuing, they would just fall out of the air after a moment of suspension.

This was not the case with me. There was no suspension time. The front tire hit the end of the roof, and the bike was now at a 90-degree angle, plummeting toward the earth like a rocket re-entry from the atmosphere. I was looking straight down at the ground, still believing that it would turn out okay.

Moments later, as I lay on the grass looking up at the sky, I noticed that the bike was suspended about a third of the way down, as if those massive tree arms chose it instead of me to save. As I lay there, my body aching, I relived my journey and the experience of hitting every single tree limb—the very limbs that we had to maneuver our bikes through each exhausting day.

My friends came scampering down the tree like squirrels after nuts to my aid, or so I thought. Turns out, it was every man for themselves, and they were NOT sticking around to take the rap for this one. Surprisingly, I only had a few bruises and a slight concussion. No broken bones. I still believe to this day that I could have succeeded in the endeavor, if only I had more momentum.

I was quite the hellion as a child. I thought myself a pretty good chemist, too. My friend across the street from me had an older brother and they made the run over the state line for illegal fireworks. Some of the best forbidden fruits were disguised as M-80's. Several aluminum garbage cans met their fate at our hands. We soon ran out of M-80's and decided we could make them ourselves. We gathered some cardboard cylinders that were about the same size as an M-80, some quarters, glue, gunpowder, and fuses.

A few duds and some minor adjustments later, and we had several pretty good sticks of dynamite. We graduated from garbage cans to dirt hills in the subdivision that was still under construction.

As you know, there is always bigger and better with teenaged boys and their toys.

We decided we wanted to see just how loud the big boom would be if we dropped the freshly minted stick down the manhole on our street. This was also our first experience with methane gas. One of my friends was chosen to be the one to drop the bomb down the hole in the lid over the manhole. As he did this, we all backed up a safe distance—you know, at least three or four feet—to watch. We waited for the explosion, and nothing happened.

We waited a little longer and still nothing. We stood there in disappointment, wondering amongst ourselves if we could get that lid off to retrieve our last bomb and try it again. Just then, we heard the much anticipated *'BOOM'* and watched as the lid came dislodged and blew off miles into the air (in actuality it was about 1 ½ or two feet) followed by a large ball of glowing fire. The ground beneath our feet shook, and we took off on a dead run to the backyard, which was quite a ways away.

We thought for sure we were in trouble, but not a word was spoken from any of our parents or neighbors. I remember there was a rumor of a slight earthquake, though. They even blamed the Air Force Base thinking they must have been doing some testing. We couldn't wait to do this again, only at night, because the fireball would be awesome! But this ended up being our last experience with methane gas and our last supply of gunpowder…for a while.

As a young man, one of the greatest experiences I had was being part of the scouting program. It was a great way to learn and grow, and I always looked forward to going to the meetings, outings, and other scouting rituals. It was one of the places where I could be with my friends, act like myself and not worry about my father.

I had several different scout leaders, and all of them were dedicated to helping us as impressionable young boys to succeed. One took us boating, water skiing, hiking and camping. He was an avid outdoorsman, and he understood how to hunt and fish. He taught us how to live off the land. He was the first to introduce me to this concept. Another had land and horses. He would take us to his property and teach us how to ride and proper horse etiquette.

We learned how to take good care of the beautiful animals and get them to trust us, and us them. This made me very excited because my father always had horses and loved them. At times it was all he talked about, and I thought that it would give us something in common. It worked partially because it gave me something to ask him that he was very knowledgeable about. But it also proved how much I didn't know, and he was quick to point that out.

We would camp at the property and get up the next morning and ride and take care of the horses, and I loved it. At the time, I thought it was his way of getting them taken care of for free, because we were brushing and feeding them, cleaning out the stables and hauling hay. However, now I cherish all that he taught us about those noble animals, because it has helped me in my everyday life and my dealings with people.

Horses are extremely intelligent and intuitive animals. They know your intentions sometimes even before you do. I grew very close to a few of them, and it was as if we were of one mind at times. I learned how to read people and trust my instincts more, simply by being around them. I cherished the time I was able to spend at 'the farm' as we affectionately called it.

One weekend we spent the first part of the day setting up the tents and campsite, and the second part of the day with the horses. It was common to spend the night at the farm so we could get as much time in as possible.

When it got dark, we would sit around a campfire and tell stories and laugh, and it was as if I had stepped out of my life and into an alternate universe where there weren't any bad things. This thought, however, was about to change, and the universe would show me exactly who was in charge.

For anyone who is not familiar with horses and how they're kept, the farm was a large piece of property—about 50 acres—and as a young boy, it seemed huge. The horses were allowed to roam the property; they had a stable which was a big barn-like structure but missing a wall on one of the sides so the horses could enter and exit freely. This gave them shelter from storms and warmth in the winter.

All around the property was a fence, not a typical fence like you see in subdivisions or urban areas, but a barbed wire fence that was about five feet tall. Now, if you know anything about horses, you know that they can leap over a five-foot fence of barbed wire just as easily as you can step over a crack in the sidewalk, so to deter them, an electric fence is used.

These fences consist of a tiny strand of wire that's connected to an energizer which sends a current of electricity through the wire. It delivers a sudden, sharp spark. The horses quickly learn where they can and where they cannot venture. All it takes is a few brushes against that wire, and being intelligent animals, they learn to look but not to touch.

I did learn about electric fences, but not through reading and setting them up, or by warnings from the scoutmaster. Although that would have been very useful.

That night at the farm we went to bed relatively early because we were planning on getting up early the next morning to hunt geese. It was October, so it was chilly but not freezing out, so sleeping in tents as long as you were bundled up wasn't bad.

Sometime in the early morning hours, I needed to relieve myself. At the farm there aren't any bathrooms, at least not formal bathrooms. So we would just walk over next to a tree or behind the stable and take care of our business.

However, at zero dark thirty in the A.M., no one can see you, so I just walked away from the tents and started doing my business. As I began, I vaguely remember a dazzling flash of light and then it all went dark. My scout mates woke up a while later and realized I was nowhere to be found. The scout leaders and the scouts started a search for me. The next thing I remember is my friends laughing and shaking me to wake me up. I was lying on the grass unconscious.

The electric fence had pulsed as I was relieving myself and unbeknownst to me, I was right next to it. In fact, I was close enough to be peeing right on it. Now many people have relayed to me how they have themselves peed on an electric fence. I have heard everything about how bad it hurt, how they peed blood and other fairly mild descriptions.

When people relay these stories, I take it at face value that it is exactly that—a story. After living through that experience, it's hard for me to just say it hurt...a lot, even. In most cases I just look at them and say, *"If all you can say is 'it hurt, like getting kicked in the balls', you're a liar!"* It seems there are a lot of variances in people's experiences, especially one:

Numerous stories involve the same type of beginning, not knowing the fence was there and then being very surprised when they found out. But the biggest difference is the fact that they were all wearing shoes or boots with rubber soles. This insulated them from the ground and thereby didn't allow the circuit to be completed.

So although they received a shock, it wasn't able to return, as current is designed to do. I, however, was sleeping, therefore I had bare feet as I walked out of the tent and into the dew covered grass, thus creating the perfect conductor—water on both ends and me in between.

The electricity entered my body and exited through my feet and into the ground. The shock, thank God, was only a tenth of a second long, but that was enough. It scorched the bottom of both of my feet and everything in between as the current exited my body.

I was taken to the hospital and would like to say it was embarrassing, but the pain I felt in my body counteracted any other feelings I may have had. I was a young teenage boy burned at both ends and in between. I was also covered in urine because, as I learned, once I started and electricity got involved, two things had happened. First, I lost consciousness and fell to the ground, thanks to the pulse action of the fence.

Second, I just continued to empty my bladder as I lay in the grass. Being in the hospital, I had my first, and I wish I could say only, experience with a catheter. The catheter served a couple of purposes; it kept my bladder empty so that it could heal from the burn that the electricity created and it held my urethra open and free from blood clots for the same reason. I later learned that there are different settings as to the intensity of the fences pulse, and the doctor believed that it was up to the maximum.

Now, I also wish I could say that I didn't feel like a magnet for shit that could go wrong. However, my life has always been one disaster after another. Just to add insult to injury, when the nurse was removing the catheter, neither she nor I was prepared for the next part. There is a small balloon type bubble on the bladder side of the catheter to keep it in place. She deflated that balloon, however, the injury to my urethra created scabbing and that scabbing adhered to the catheter.

As the catheter was removed, it pulled the scabs off the inside of my urinary tract sending me into excruciating pain and causing bleeding once again. They monitored me for several days to make sure that surgery wouldn't be necessary and to ensure that no other problems ensued.

I still suffer several other side effects from this experience, one of them being regulation of body temperature, as my ability to feel cold or hot was diminished. I had to learn just to stay warm in the winter and cool in the summer whether I felt it or not.

Other things were also affected; the hormones from the hypothalamus govern physiologic functions such as thirst, hunger, sleep, mood, sex drive, and the release of other hormones within the body. All of these have been an issue my entire life.

The age I wasn't expected to see grew with every birthday. As you can tell, I made it past all of them. But my mom had plenty of reasons to worry.

11
I Punched Him Sober

*"Experience: that most brutal of teachers.
But you learn, my God do you learn."*

— C. S. Lewis

As a teenage boy, I was still searching for what would define me as an adult. However, with the relationship I had with my father, I chose to follow a path of *'I WILL SHOW YOU!'* This can go one of two ways; one being the road to change and doing the best I possibly could to show him I was worth something. Or the other; since you already believe that I am so bad I might as well be bad. I, of course, chose the latter.

My self-esteem was at an all-time low. I searched for a place to belong. I found myself following the wrong crowd of people early on. My 'friends' all ended up in jail or prison for one reason or another. And I, probably through divine intervention, seemed always to know when they were headed in the 'wrong direction' and bailed before I also ended up there.

I was never really like them and didn't participate in several the actions of my friends. I just needed something that provided me with the title of 'troublemaker' and a feeling of belonging. Or so I thought. I felt that I was in it for the recognition. Like I said, I was going to be *something*, and at this point, it was going to be America's Most Wanted. My dad, seeing what was happening to me, decided to step into my path and try to help…but in his way, which was and wasn't the best thing for me.

The action taken by my dad did two things for me in my life. First, it gave me the direction that I so wanted and needed in my life. Second, it started me on the path that led me to where I am now.

My father signed me up for martial arts.

Martial arts provided a couple of things that I was lacking. In the beginning, it was a way to get out some built up aggression, due to the constant emotional beating I received from my father. It also started building my self-esteem. However, the self-esteem that I was building wasn't necessarily moving me in the right direction.

As you can probably guess, I used it to fight my way to 'respect.' I use the term respect in the way I saw it back then. I became my father, fighting with anyone who would say the wrong thing or look at me the wrong way. I learned very fast that fighting was something I was good at—probably too good—and I used it to satisfy my desire for acceptance.

For years, I carried on this way. I was fighting my way deeper and deeper into a personal hole of mental and emotional distress. But eventually, I found the father that I was missing in my Sensei, Tyrone. He took me on as his personal project, and we found something that we both needed; I found a male role model who showed me love and compassion. And he found someone he could teach and raise as a son.

This arrangement created a very positive environment for me and channeled my fighting into point tournaments and the full contact ring. I learned that the things in life that mattered most were those that made a difference in someone else's life. The little things that Tyrone did for me that had no direct effect on him but made my life better, showed me that life's best gifts are those that you give to others.

The positive environment of the dojo changed my life. I went from a misguided boy fighting to gain 'respect' to an esteemed Sensei in my own right. My students were taught with the same love and honor that my Sensei showed me. And from then on, every person I met, I treated with the respect that I so longed for as a young man. A wise person knows that there is something to be gleaned from everyone. I learned that every person I came in contact with had something to teach me.

Thanks to this, I was able to experience things that I would never have been able to, if I would have stayed on the path that I was following. My journey to what I now share and believe started here with the opening of my mind, heart, and soul. I realized that life had more to offer than any other formal opportunity that I had for the rest of my life.

I received my black belt February 19th, 1988. That same year was the first year that Tae-Kwon-Do was introduced into the Olympics in Seoul, Korea. It was classified as a demonstration sport but it was exciting just the same. I tried out for the Olympic team. However, I was trained as a full contact fighter and not a point fighter. There are a lot of differences, the biggest being that, in point fighting, you make little to no contact with your opponent. In full contact—well, that's self-explanatory. Even though I didn't make the team, our dojo, including my Sensei and I, was appointed to the AAU, which stands for the Amateur Athletic Union.

This is the governing body for the Olympics. This was a great honor for me, as I became one of the instructors for those competing in the Olympics.

I had been training very hard up to this point in my life. I was spending four hours a night, five nights a week at the dojo. This was everything to me, and all of my so-called friends that were going down the wrong path had been excluded from my life.

I credit my martial arts and my Sensei for this. It was the love of the martial arts, the love of the feeling of being in shape, strong and powerful in my mind and body that allowed me to break free from their influence. It was also martial arts that allowed me to

I PUNCHED HIM SOBER

decline all of the offers of drugs or other harmful substances or experiences.

I trained very hard and was proud of what I had become. As all martial artists, I admired the great Bruce Lee. He had perfected what was called a one-inch punch. I worked for hundreds of hours on duplicating the punch. By no means did I compare to Bruce Lee, however, I did become quite proficient in my own right.

I also worked very hard and became proficient at the free falling board break. This technique is holding a 12 inch square pine board at eye level, then releasing the board, bringing that same hand back to your chest and, as quickly as possible, striking the board as it falls to the ground with enough energy to break the board. This is tough to do because there is no support for the board as there is in traditional breaking.

These particular techniques became quite popular at demonstrations and tournaments. Several of my friends had heard of this and wished me to demonstrate it for them. One of these instances was with one of my good friends, Chris.

I was working as a D.J. for high school and college dances as well as corporate and private events part-time. Chris was one of the full-time D.J.s who worked for the same company. He and I quickly became great friends and we worked together almost every weekend for several years. When I first met Chris, he was 12 years old, but his knowledge of music and mixing was the best I had ever seen.

After a couple of years together, we were doing a dance for the University of Utah in Salt Lake City. We were setting up massive amounts of sound equipment and lighting in a gigantic ballroom where thousands of college students were coming to have a good time. We arrived in enough time that we got our lighting, sound and video screens all set up about an hour before the dance.

Chris and I sat on a bench at the rear of the ballroom and talked as we usually did. He was very curious about my martial arts background. We were discussing the one-inch punch, its philosophy, technique and the amount of power that can be generated.

Chris was skeptical, to say the least. In fact, he was downright disbelieving. He begged and begged me to demonstrate this one-inch punch, but he was only 15 years old, and me being an adult didn't bode well in my mind. Neither did trying to explain to law enforcement why I punched this kid. I was pretty sure that the police wouldn't believe that he begged me to hit him.

After about 15 minutes of him berating me with his cynicism, I complied. We were sitting on a bench that was wide enough for the two of us with about 18 inches of space in between us. He was on my left side, and I simply raised my left hand up to his shoulder and extended my fingers until the tips of my fingers just touched his shoulder, with my arm bent at the elbow there was only barely enough room to do this. I closed my fingers into a fist and in the same instant moved my fist forward to his shoulder with just enough energy to knock him off the end of the bench, landing on his butt on the hard marble floor. Needless to say, Chris never doubted that punch, or me, ever again.

Many years later, Chris and I were both at a party with mutual friends. He, in his slightly intoxicated state, was bragging about my one-inch punch and how much energy I could produce. Once again, he begged for a demonstration to prove to our friends how powerful it was. Our friends were as disbelieving as he was several years ago when I first showed it to him.

Now, I had been drinking and was not in a proper state of mind, However, as we all know, when you have been drinking, all logic goes right out the window. I finally gave in and proceeded to demonstrate the punch for all of our friends in attendance.

Chris planted both his feet on the grass in a wide stance to give him as much balance and stability as possible. He put his arms to his sides and puffed out his chest, tightening up all his torso muscles in preparation. I should also mention at this point that when alcohol is involved, not only was logic out the window, but so was my ability to control the energy that I used in this punch.

I planted my feet, squared my hips, and placed my fingers on Chris's sternum. I asked him if he was ready and he stated, *"Hell yeah, let's do this!"* I closed my fingers, and before anyone could blink, Chris was flying through the air backward. It looked as if he had an invisible rope tied around his waist and the other end attach to a car that had just slammed the accelerator to the floor.

His arms and feet shot straight out in front of him as he flew back about eight feet, once again landing flat on his butt and sliding through the grass another two to three feet. Everyone at the party was immediately silent, and I realized at that point I may have just severely injured, if not killed, one of my best friends.

My daughter was at this party with us. She was not drinking because she was the best drunk-adult babysitter ever. After Chris had picked himself up, my daughter ran over to him to make sure he was okay and that nothing was broken. After brushing him off and talking to him for a little while just to make sure that everything was fine, she turned to me and said, *"Dad, I think you punched him sober."*

That was the first time any of my friends had ever witnessed my use of any of my knowledge of martial arts. I'm glad that no one was severely injured in the process, and I'm glad that my friendship with Chris stayed intact. We are still very close; we hunt and fish together and we sometimes still drink together and talk about that night. However, he has never asked me to demonstrate it again.

As I was progressing through the ranks of martial arts, it seemed that I had to work harder and that I struggled more than a lot of the students. I just didn't have the energy. My muscles would give out, and I would have to sit and rest for a while when all of the other students could continue. This frustrated me to no end, and it made me work harder.

Looking back, I recognize the symptomatology of this disease and how it was affecting me even back then. I learned that I needed to keep going no matter what the pain or fatigue level was and not let it win.

An energy failure disorder is just that—energy failure. As a young man, I didn't understand, but that's exactly what was happening to me. The production of energy in my body would just stop. A profound example of this was when I was competing professionally.

Before the popularity of the MMA fighting, there was Professional Kickboxing Association or P.K.A. This was a full contact karate match in a ring just like boxing; only both hands and feet were used.

The object is to either strike your opponent enough times to win the match or knock out your opponent. In one of these particular events, I experienced one of the worst energy failures I had in my life. There are 12 two-minute rounds. We were in the third round, and up until this point I was winning, but the match was very close.

At about 50 seconds into the third round, my legs decided that they did not want to work anymore. The only way I can describe this feeling is that an anesthetic had been injected into both of my legs. It was so powerful that they didn't even have enough strength to hold up my body weight. I just collapsed in the middle of the ring. The referee immediately stopped the fight and came over to me. I was trying to plead my case that I was fine, even though I couldn't stand or walk, but he stopped the fight, declaring my opponent the winner by technical knockout.

Paramedics responded to the ring. However, after several minutes the energy had returned and I was able to stand and walk and move around. That was one of the most embarrassing and challenging days of my life. I had trained so hard. I had all of the advantages except the disorder that was hiding inside of me of which I was unaware.

I started teaching martial arts, when a middle-aged man became a new student. We quickly became friends. He was a professor at a local college, and he started my formal education by enrolling me in school.

This was not an easy process, as I only achieved six credits throughout my high school years. I wasn't the brightest crayon in the box, so getting scholarships was laughable. He helped me fill out the paperwork for admission, as well as all the grant and funding papers. He vouched for me that he would personally guarantee my attendance and grades, basically begging the school to admit me.

I graduated from adult high school with honors, and I received my first college degree with his help. He spent hours tutoring me and mentoring me throughout my schooling. During this time, I was also up for my Black Belt testing. The Masters were coming to witness the trial—I had the knowledge, but I wasn't ready.

He took time daily at his lunch hour to watch me prepare for my Black Belt testing. Once again, here was a man who was willing to sacrifice his own time for a young man who was trying to find his way in life. Although he was an excellent professor and teacher of curriculum, he taught me that above all,

"The most important learning one can receive is from one's experiences."

We remained friends, and I was proud and honored to be the Sensei that promoted and presented him his Black Belt just a few short years later. The time and love that he showed me I could never repay, but being there and honoring him with that achievement will always be one of my most memorable experiences.

12
TIME TO BE A MAN

"Be the person you needed when you were younger."

— *Unknown*

I always cry at military funerals. It doesn't matter whose funeral it is, just knowing the sacrifice that they made for us and this country always seems to bring out that emotional response. Several times I have attended a funeral for a distant relative or another person with whom I have no real emotional ties. Once Taps start, I start crying like a schoolgirl looking at a positive pregnancy test. Of all the military funerals I've ever attended, there is one that stands out in my mind, and always will.

When My Uncle Terry came into my life, I was in my adolescence. I didn't realize how much impact he would have on me and how much of him I would incorporate into my life. He tried to do everything that he could to help me and to teach me how to treat people and earn respect. He was career military, worked very hard in the Air Force and retired as a Master Sergeant. Clearly, he understood what it took to make a man. He was the first adult family member to show me the same respect that he would show any of his colleagues. For many years, he was another of my pseudo-fathers.

Out of the three men who mentored me, this was the man that I spent the most time with one on one. He and my aunt did not have children of their own, and he was close enough to my situation to know that I needed guidance. He took me on hunting and fishing trips that gave us the opportunity to bond. He was a highly educated man and also very knowledgeable about life and the importance of experience. It was this education that he passed on to me.

My father could never admit his wrongs. It was like a personal attack on his character. Throughout my life, my father would always find blame and fault in someone else. I don't think I ever heard my father say he was wrong. It was always my fault and then, when I grew old enough to argue, it was my kids, cousins or later in life, some made-up random person that he created.

This trait was passed down to me, as I learned through watching him, over and over, that this was how blame should be placed. For many years, I had the same way of responding to failures. I placed blame on others and I never admitted fault, no matter the evidence against me. I also believe that my search for acceptance caused me to think that if I were wrong, that would make me less of a person and, therefore, people wouldn't want to be around me. My father had made it very clear that no one wants to associate with someone who isn't right all the time.

My uncle allowed me to make mistakes and, unlike my father, he would use those mistakes as opportunities to teach. He would talk to me and show me the careless ways in which I acted at times or the errors that I may have made. Rather than beat me down as a disgraceful and embarrassing child, he used them to show me the proper way and was the first person to teach me to accept my mistakes and learn from them in order to make my life better.

He showed me that he didn't like it when he made a mistake, but that it was a part of life and a part of growing up. He didn't often need correcting, but when he did, he would face up to it, take responsibility and offer a solution or, at least, a sincere apology.

I always looked up to my uncle; he seemed to be such a large man, and he was always in control. He always had answers and suggestions for any issues that might arise.

My first experience with my uncle was as a very young boy. At the time, my family consisted of my two older sisters, me and a younger sister who was only a year old. We went to visit my uncle in Colorado when he was stationed at the Air Force Academy. He took my dad and me sightseeing while the girls went about their day. I vividly remember visiting Santa's workshop at the North Pole, which mysteriously was close to the Air Force Base.

North Pole Colorado is a Christmas-themed amusement park, but being four or five, I didn't know any better; I was just excited to meet Santa and the elves. This was the time that I was most hyper and now, looking back, I can see that it irritated my uncle because he was so used to the order of the military. He saw me as undisciplined and without focus, just like many other people saw me.

Years later, after he retired, he and my aunt Carol—my dad's sister—returned to Utah to live. He was from Texas, but my aunt wanted to be back with her family here in Utah. She said she had traveled long enough and wanted to be home, so they moved a short distance from my parents.

It took several years before he attempted to help me, but when he stepped in, it was worth the wait. I saw him several times over the years; fishing, hunting, at birthdays or Christmas. In the beginning, he would say or do things in an attempt to help me grow, but I was young and didn't see what he was doing. When I became a teenager, he decided it was time. At first, it was just a few simple suggestions like shaking hands, how to do it correctly—firm but not so firm that it hurt the other individual. Then it progressed to spending weekend nights at their house. It was these times that he spent discussing how a young man should act, not only around him, but in public and around everyone if I wished to gain respect.

As I grew older, we spent more and more time in the great outdoors together. He taught me the correct way to ask permission in a respectful manner. I remember spending hours on the bank of a river or a lake, catching fish and doing what I believed to be telling stories.

But as I look back, I realize that everything we did was his way of teaching me life lessons. We spent year after year hunting deer in the Wasatch Mountains; he would take me along as we hiked, rather than me being with my father. As we would sit and watch for deer, being quiet and patient was a necessity. He spent years teaching me that quality. Going through this disorder and all of the other trials of my life, having patience and being able to sit quiet and process things in my mind is one of the most valuable tools—the greatest gift—he taught me.

Even though I wasn't really into sports, he was. I didn't know much about them, but he did his best to teach me and to include me in the games that he would watch. When I was in my early teens, we started a rivalry in football. Being from Texas and growing up just outside of the Dallas area, he was an adamant Dallas Cowboys fan. I decided at that point that my favorite team in football was going to be, well, whoever was playing *against* the Dallas Cowboys. This wasn't to mock him or hurt him, and there was no malice or animosity between the two of us; it was just my friendly way to be part of the game.

He would talk for hours about the team, the players and all of the advancements that they used to keep them safe. He tried his hardest to get me to become a Dallas fan. However the harder he tried, the harder I pushed back. I made sure I knew what team was playing Dallas that week, then I would call and make friendly wagers on the game. He knew that it was all in good fun; however, I do believe it still got to him just a little bit that I wouldn't turn to the dark side with him.

To this day, my favorite NFL football team is whoever is playing the Dallas Cowboys. It has nothing to do with not liking that team. It keeps his memory alive in me, the rivalry and fun that we had. Keeping that little bit of him still within me, knowing that he would appreciate that I never backed down or changed my favorite team. It was always more important to him that I stood behind my convictions and beliefs, rather than following along with someone else. I believe he always knew that my rivalry with him and the Cowboys was just my way of joining him in something that he loved.

When it came to some of the more negative things in life, he taught me how to make correct decisions. For example, he smoked from the time he was a teenager. I remember as we spent days together I would count the number of cigarettes that he would smoke in a day. I even got to the point where I would count the number of breaths that it took for him to exhale the smoke out of his lungs. I hated that he did this. I talked to him about it and tried to discourage him, but he turned it into a lesson as well.

"Don't ever start, because once you do, it's just too hard to quit!" or *"This was the stupidest thing I've ever done in my life."* He always made sure that I understood that it wasn't cool or sophisticated or anything more than a bad choice. He tried several times to quit but, again, looking back, I can see that he did enjoy it for whatever reason. For him it was just part of his life. My aunt finally quit after years of trying, but my uncle never did.

We continued to hunt and fish together, and he continued to help me along on my journey to becoming the person that I am today. I visited him every chance I got, and we would talk and discuss daily life. When I was in my early twenties, he told me that he was getting to a point in his life where he could no longer go hunting as much as we had been.

He offered to sell me his rifle that he used all of those years, and I jumped at the opportunity to own that piece of our time together. I hunted with his rifle for many years, and every year it felt as if he was right there with me—my uncle, by my side, still there to guide and direct me—keeping me on the path.

After several years of spending time together, my uncle pulled me aside to tell me that when he first met me those many years ago in Colorado, and then after moving to Utah, he believed that I was a lost cause. As a young man, he thought I was undisciplined and arrogant and was never going to amount to anything in life.

He then told me that he was wrong, that he was proud of me and that I had turned into a fine, upstanding, respectful young man. There has never been another time in my life when an individual has said anything to me that has meant as much as that statement from him.

A few short years later, my mentor and uncle was diagnosed with cancer. In very little time, cancer, radiation, chemotherapy and all of the other medical procedures he had to go through transformed that strong, powerful man into a withered shell. It was tough for me to visit him during this time. I regret that more than any other regrets I have in my life—I wasn't there for him in his time of need. It hurt me so bad to see him in that condition, and I wanted to remember him as the strong, powerful man that he was.

I never got the opportunity to repay him for all of the things that he taught me and helped me with in life. I know I was wrong not to visit him while he was sick as much as I should have. I went fishing with him a few more times, and I saw him at his home once or twice, but I was a very foolish person…still wanting what I used to have and not what was in front of me. As much as I loved and cherished him, as honored as I was when he told me he was proud of me, and how much he meant to me in my life, I still couldn't bring myself to see him in that way.

My aunt tried to comfort me by telling me he didn't want anybody to see him in that condition. And although I know that is true, I can't help but believe that I abandoned him.

Both my Uncle Terry and the man who put me on the path to my education have now passed on, after fighting valiant battles with cancer. Their life on this earth may be over, but for the people they touched with love, respect, and genuine caring, they will never be forgotten. As long as I have breath, their inspiration will never be lost. They are a huge part of who I am and what I aspire to be in my life. Rest In Peace, and thank you for teaching me the most important things in life aren't always what we expect them to be, but rather what we make of the unexpected.

13
SAVED BY AN ANGEL

*"You will not be punished for your anger;
you will be punished by your anger."*

— *Buddha*

There are many things in my life that I am incredibly proud of. One of those is the fact that I have gone my entire life without ever experimenting with any illegal substances. That isn't to say that some of my closest friends, those that I hung out with every day, could also say that.

In junior high and high school, I was surrounded by the drug culture and heavy drug use. Even though there were a lot of drugs out there, the one that I saw most was marijuana. Several of my friends had at least experimented with it and some were regular users. My friends and I had an agreement; I didn't partake, and they didn't push the issue or try to pressure me into trying anything. Basically because they knew I could beat the shit out of them if they did.

This didn't mean that I didn't have other vices that were just as detrimental, if not more. I want you to understand that I am not proud or bragging about the following incidents; this was just a vital intersection in my life. Some of these things I regretted for a very long time until I realized that they were lessons to be learned. It was a time when I needed to get over the issues I was struggling with in life and with my father, and to be young. I didn't have the ability to logically figure out a more productive way of doing that.

When I was in junior high, I had been in martial arts for about three years. It was during this time when I was abundantly angry and vengeful. I was well known as a person to stay away from.

I wasn't afraid to fight, no matter who I might have been up against. I was also very reckless in a lot of other ways. I was suspended or expelled from school several times because of altercations. There were two particular times that I look back on now, wishing I would have learned some of those lessons in a different way. But I realize it had to be learned, and this was just how it happened.

I was about 14 years old, and I was in art class. As usual, I was probably messing around, acting out and doing things I absolutely should not have been doing in class. It was a time when teachers were still allowed to discipline students. Not necessarily physical punishment, but they didn't have to worry about the lawsuits of today.

The classroom teacher walked up behind me, and he grabbed my left arm and my shoulder to spin me around, more than likely as a means of getting my attention and instructing me to either finish my assignment or leave his classroom.

I immediately rolled my left arm over the top of his locking him in an armbar as I spun to face him. I grabbed his throat with my right hand, squeezing just enough to make him choke and gag. I walked him backward until he was up against the wall and very forcefully advised him, "Never touch me again. Next time I will tear your throat out." Needless to say, I was expelled from school. For some unknown reason, though, the school district felt it was unnecessary to press charges.

The second time was a year later; I was in ninth grade when my father was committed for a psychiatric evaluation for the first time. He lost control at work after being denied a promotion and he proceeded to tear the furniture apart, break windows and attack anything and anybody in his path. (People often wondered where I got my anger from.)

On this particular day, my mother called the school and told me that he had been taken to the hospital and that she wouldn't be there to pick me up after school; I was to go home with my cousin and stay there until she got home. I was so elated and excited about my father's commitment that, as I was walking down the hallway, I was jumping up and kicking the lockers.

As I was doing this, one of the teachers heard me in the hall, came out and grabbed me by the back of my neck. I spun and punched him three times in the face before I even realized that it was a teacher. He dropped to the floor, blood streaming from his nose and lip. Before I could even apologize or explain my actions, I was, once again, down in the office being expelled from school.

I got into many fights during this time of my life, for any reasons I could muster. I had the idea that people should respect me. And if they didn't, they would learn to. My anger controlled me; it was as if that was the fuel for my engine, my driving force. It was the one thing that I knew I was good at. In fact, I was exceptional, and I used that knowledge to what I believed was my advantage.

It didn't matter if it was in school, after school or even during the summer break. In fact, when I was only 15 years old, I was stabbed in a fight. I was on an anger walk one evening after having an argument with my dad. My anger walks were supposed to calm me down, but they didn't always work.

During my walk, I confronted two older boys that were snickering about how I was dressed; I was wearing hand-me-downs from my sisters. I immediately started verbally berating the two boys, and they were not about to be talked to that way by someone two or three years younger than them. They came over to me, puffing out their chests to intimidate me, and started pushing me and calling me names. I did have some form of what I believed was honor, so I allowed them to shove me three or four times before I reacted. This made it self-defense in my mind.

This was also an excellent fighting tactic because it always caught them off guard. If I allowed them to push me two or three times, and acted afraid, they began thinking they had the advantage, and they wouldn't see the strikes coming.

I only weighed about 150 pounds, but I was fast as lightning. In this case, one of the boys was larger than the other, and I knew it would take longer to put him down. I also knew that if the larger of the two was taken out first, there was a good chance the other one would just back down, and I wouldn't have to fight both of them. I started hitting the first boy, and I made contact with every strike.

This, however, was a mistake; I misread the two individuals. I threw a barrage of punches and kicks at the first boy, and he fell right to the ground covering his head and face, trying to protect himself. He never even attempted to punch me back. I immediately turned to face the second boy in hopes that he would be backing away, but to my surprise he was swinging at me as I turned. What I didn't notice was the knife he was holding.

As I parried his punch, the knife veered away from my chest, cutting a slice in my shirt and about two inches across the top of my shoulder. Instinctively, I grabbed his arm and broke it between his wrist and elbow. As I heard the bones snap, the pain was too much, and he released the knife. I proceeded to kick him several times in the ribs and face and then pushed him to the ground next to his friend. I picked up the knife and both of them stood and ran. There were several other times I was involved in a fight with a knife. No one was ever killed, but there were always injuries.

Not only was fighting my way to release anger, so was acting up and getting in trouble. At times, I would do things on purpose just to get caught, to get in trouble and be punished, because I felt that's what I should be—punished. It also meant my father suffered humiliation every time I was brought home, or he had to pick me up after I was caught doing something wrong. I had been told my entire life that I was a disappointment and a failure, so I was trying to live up to that title.

In ninth grade, during gym class, we would get dressed and go out onto the football field where the gym teacher would meet us, take roll and then we would play flag football.

The only real upside to gym class was the girls would also come out and line up on their side, right in front of all of us guys, to wait for their gym teacher. They would then go off and play softball or other activities at the opposite end of the field.

One particular fall morning the boys were all lined up outside of the gym locker room, waiting for the teacher to come out. That's when I had the most brilliant of ideas, and I convinced them to follow my plan. It was simple; we'd all stand in line and wait for the girl's class to come outside, and then every one of the guys would turn, drop their shorts, and moon the girls.

We were laughing and giggling like young teenage boys do, thinking we were so hilarious, but no good deed goes unpunished. At the very moment that we dropped our shorts—all 32 of us showing our bare assets for the entire world to see—both gym teachers exited the building.

The punishment that we received for this act wasn't administrative or suspension. Our gym teacher simply made us run the bleachers for the entire class period every day for two full weeks. Even being in great shape, not knowing about my disorder at the time made running those bleachers tough. Several times I tripped and fell, bruising and scraping up my shins. I felt as if my legs were made out of sand, but I kept right up with all of the other guys; after all, it was my idea.

When I got into high school, my life hadn't changed much. I was spending a lot of time with the friends that would hang out in the parking lot and smoke their pot, drink beer and avoid going to classes.

This is where another turn for the worse happened in my life. I told you that I was very proud that I never tried an illegal substance in my life, and that is true. However, that does not apply to alcohol. By my Sophomore year of high school, I spent almost every day with my friends, drinking whatever I could get my hands on.

I was usually intoxicated by nine or ten o'clock in the morning and tried to maintain that throughout the day. There were many days that I would show up in class with a Big Gulp cup that was half Coke and half some kind of whiskey. At this point, I didn't even care if I got caught. My self-esteem was the lowest it had ever been. Along with this, I withdrew from all of my friends and became angrier and more self-deprecating.

Little did I know that one of the greatest events in my life was about to happen; something that was going to change my life forever, and I almost missed it because I was drunk.

I was 16 years old and I didn't attend many classes, or on the rare occasion that I did, I would sit alone, generally in the back of a room, avoiding contact with anybody and everybody. Mostly because I was still drunk or, at least, hung over. This was one of those days.

As I sat in my chair with a headache and light sensitivity from that morning's binge, the most beautiful, spirited, friendly girl walked in and sat down right beside me. To my complete shock, she looked at me and said, *"Hey, Shawn. How are you today?"* The only thought that went through my mind was, *"Who are you and why are you talking to me?"* Then the second thought, *"How do you know my name?"*

Apparently we had met the day before, but I was so intoxicated that I didn't remember. I was in shock and awe, upset at myself because this beautiful girl remembered me, but I did not recognize her. I learned that she was dating one of my friends at the time, and he'd introduced her to me the day before, but I was working on my second or third Big Gulp and didn't have my wits about me.

I attended class two days in a row, and sober, which was new for me. I wanted to see if that young lady was real or an alcohol induced hallucination. Sure enough, the next day, she came right in and sat down next to me again and started talking to me. I remembered all of this conversation and how mesmerized I was. After about a week of attending that class just to see her, I stopped drinking.

Her name was Cindee, spelled with two E's. Up to that point in my life, she was the greatest thing that ever happened to me.

We spent an hour together every day, talking, flirting and doing anything but classwork. After a couple of months of this, she broke up with her boyfriend, and we started seeing each other regularly. We dated all through our sophomore year and that summer. I had stopped drinking altogether and even stopped hanging out with most of my friends to be with her. I was, however, still fighting.

One particular fight was defending her honor. We were at one of the high school football games during our junior year, sitting together, keeping warm under a blanket, cuddling and enjoying life. As we were sitting there, one of my friends and some of his new friends were sitting behind us, being obnoxious and drunk as usual. I had learned to ignore them, but this time, they didn't want to be ignored.

When the game was over, we left, found something to eat, and I took her home. I received a phone call from my friend who was behind us, and he told me that one of the guys with him at the game was saying a lot of derogatory things about my girlfriend. He called her some very nasty names that I will not repeat here. Some things should never be said about a woman.

I became incredibly angry, and it fueled the fire of my hatred all night. I was like a steam engine with coal being shoveled into the furnace to build heat to supply enough energy to make it over a mountain. The next morning when I got to school, I stood just down the hall from this boy's locker, waiting for him to arrive. He was shorter than me, but he was on the school wrestling and football teams and outweighed me by about 30 pounds. None of that mattered; he would have had to be a rhinoceros to exceed my anger at this point.

When he got to his locker, he saw me standing in the hall, waiting, and he laughed and sneered and said something derogatory to his friends that were with him. As I walked up to him, his friends were facing me, but his back was towards me. He was still talking, and his friends were laughing until they saw me approach.

A look of dread crossed their faces, and they started backing down the hall away from him—and me.

As he turned and saw me, he said, *"What the hell do you want?"* I never answered him; I hit him as hard as I possibly could.

I put every bit of energy that was in my body into that punch. After I had swung, he just stood there staring at me, and I thought for the first time I had bitten off more than I could chew. As I prepared to continue hitting him, his eyes rolled back in his head, and he collapsed to the floor, unconscious.

This angered me more; the fight was over too quickly. In my mind, I didn't get my fair justice. I immediately grabbed him and lifted his limp head off the floor to keep punching his unconscious face, but my friends dragged me off of him and down the hall, the whole time trying to calm me down. It took several minutes for him to regain consciousness and one of his friends ended up taking him to the hospital.

I had fractured his cheek and eye socket, and he had a concussion. Fortunately, he never required surgery or any other medical procedures. Even though the police and his parents continually questioned him about who was responsible, he never told them it was me.

I didn't graduate from high school with my class. I needed 18 credits to graduate that year and I had earned six. However, Cindee and I were continuing to grow closer and stronger. We spent all day together at school and a lot of evenings after school. She was teaching me to remain calm, and was giving me a reason to believe in myself and gain some self-worth.

I still had a lot of anger issues and, even more, self-esteem issues; but when I was with her, it was as if I was in a world where none of that negativity existed. A place where my father never existed and my anger never existed. All there was, was our love. As angry and hateful as I was, I was never angry or hateful towards her. I never raised my voice or treated her negatively in any way.

Cindee was the total opposite of me. She was a straight-A student all through elementary school and junior high. When she got into high school, she took advanced courses in English and Math, trying to prepare herself for college. She was a member of VECA and in her junior year, was accepted to be on the yearbook staff. She started working part time for a credit union.

She was the co-editor of the yearbook in our senior year and designed the cover. Cindee was the studious type, and never really struggled with homework. Things just came naturally to her, except for Trigonometry. She would try to solve the equations and get frustrated. I never took a math class higher than general math, but for whatever reason, I could look at the equation and come up with the answer. I had no idea how to go through the steps to get to the answer, but somehow, I knew it. She had the memory of an elephant. Anyone that needed a family member's phone number would ask her, and she would rattle it off as quickly and regularly as tying a shoe.

I tried several times to get Cindee to sluff a class with me, but she never did. Partly because she was afraid of getting caught, but mostly because she enjoyed school. I would pick her up in the morning, drop her off at school, then I would go and do whatever it was I did during the day. After school I would pick her up, and we would go home—usually to her house. She would quickly do her homework, then we would spend the rest of the evening together, watching TV or working on something in the garage—it didn't matter what we did, we were together.

We were very different. We were also very much the same. We shared an absolute love of the outdoors. We both enjoyed camping, fishing, and hunting. We both loved dogs and had an intense dislike for cats. We liked to laugh and spend time with friends. We also had similar tastes in food. We learned that we both liked Chinese and Mexican food. We both hated liver. I liked mushrooms, and she hated them. I liked peppers; she didn't. She liked avocados, and I wasn't that fond of them. She loved rice crispy treats and to me, they were like Kryptonite to Superman.

We were the perfect mix.

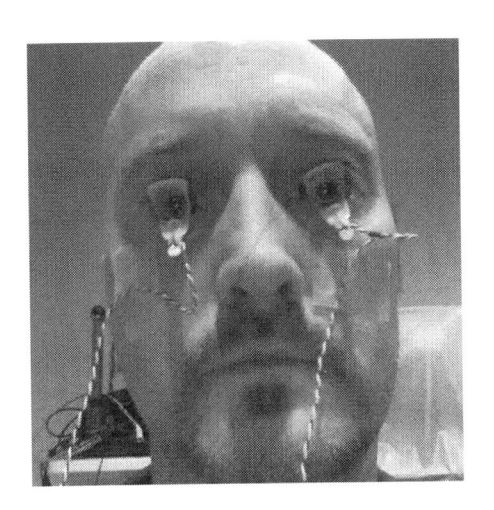

SAVED BY AN ANGEL

Metal Electrodes Attached To My Eyes.

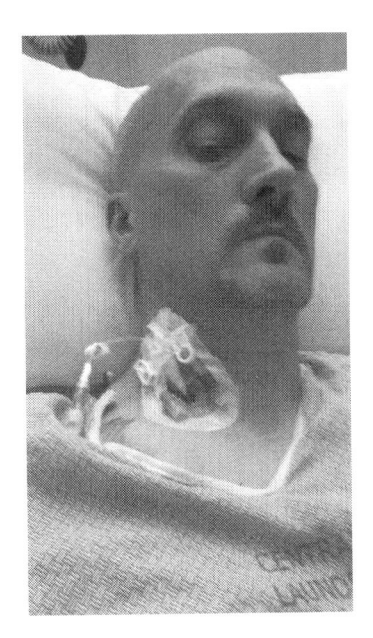

Juglar I.V. Port

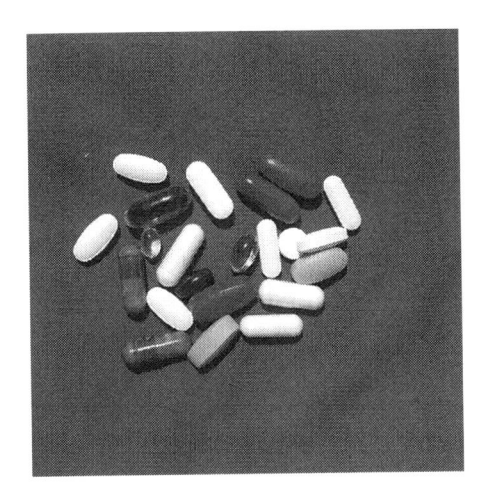

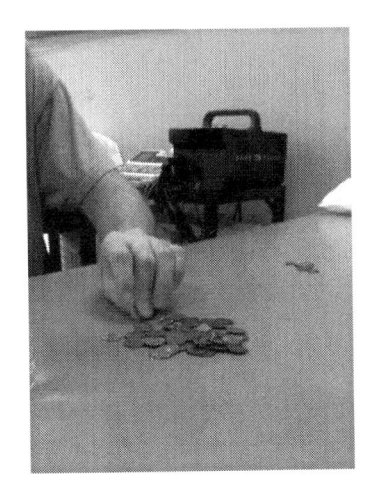

Daily Amino Acids

Relearning To Use
My Fingers

SHAWN PAULSEN

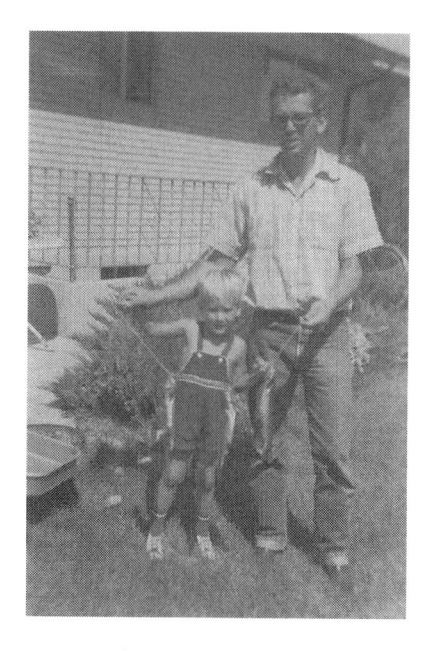

Fishing With My Dad

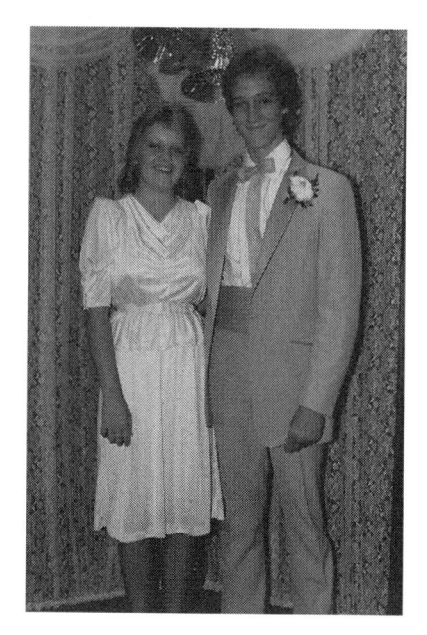

High School Days

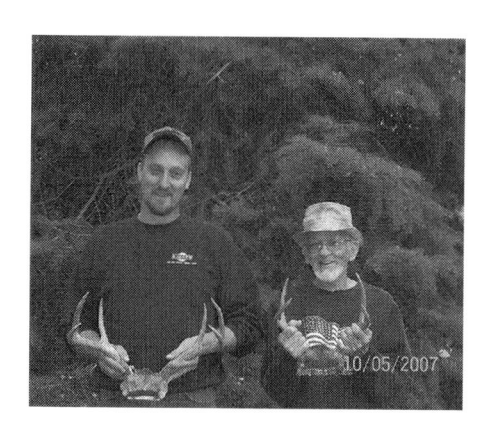

Last Hunting Trip With My Dad

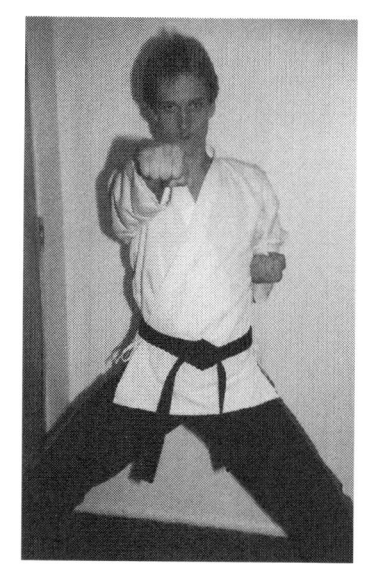

Martial Arts

SAVED BY AN ANGEL

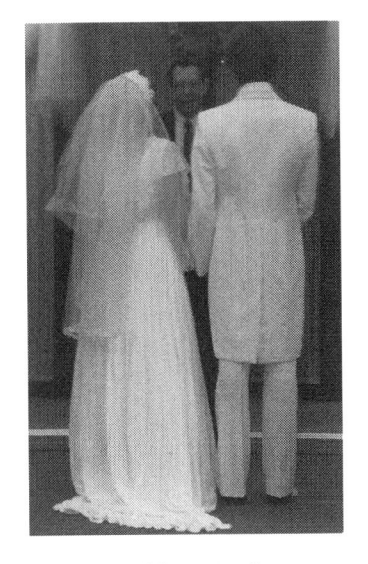

Wedding Socks

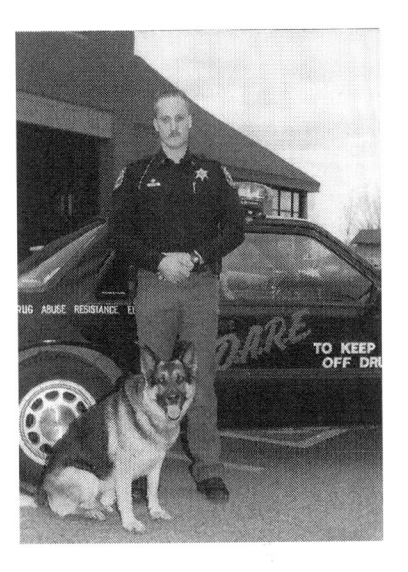

Law Enforcement With Barron

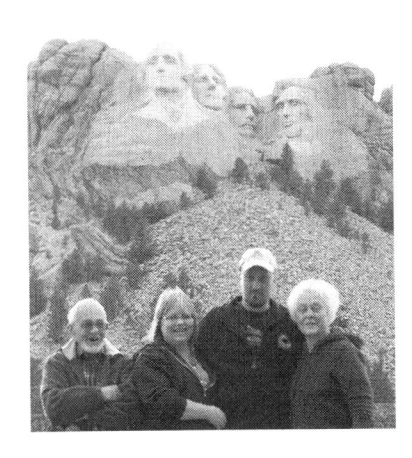

Moms First Trip To
Mt. Rushmore

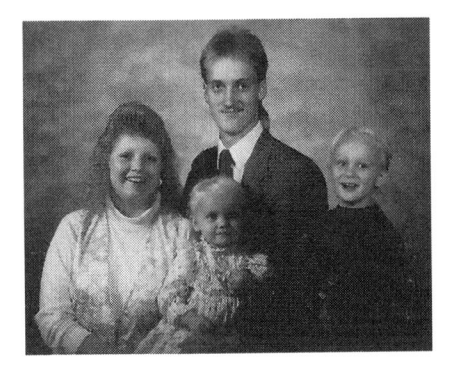

My Young Family

SHAWN PAULSEN

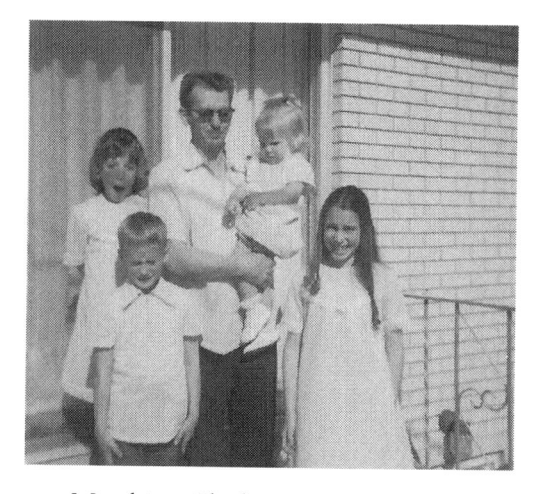

Matching Clothes My Mom Made
Approximately The Time Of The Milk Incident

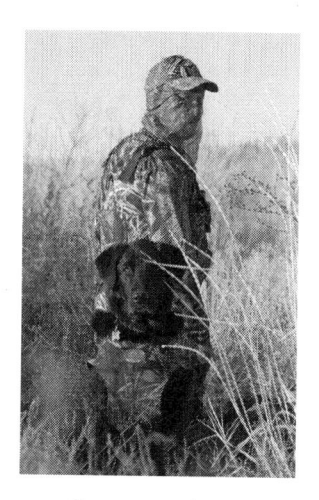

Dozer And Me

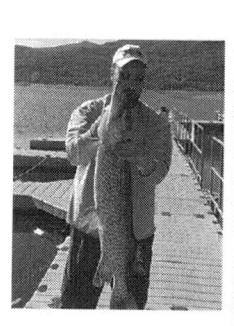

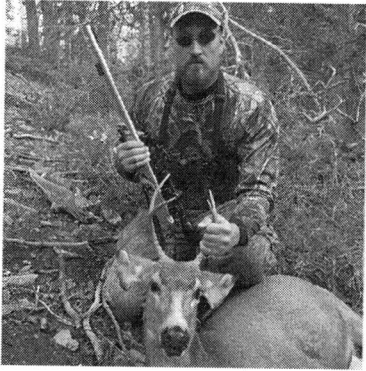

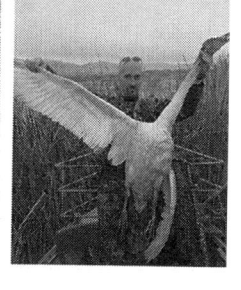

My First Deer, Swan And Muskie After Going Blind

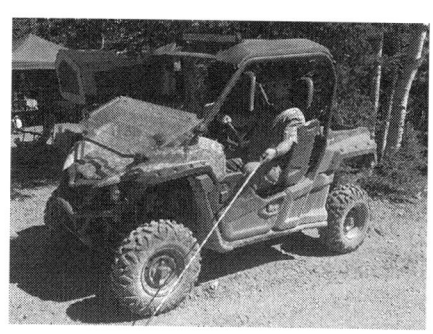

Driving The UTV With My Cane

SAVED BY AN ANGEL

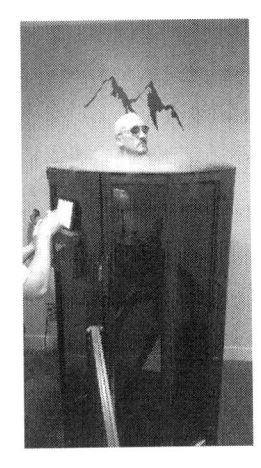

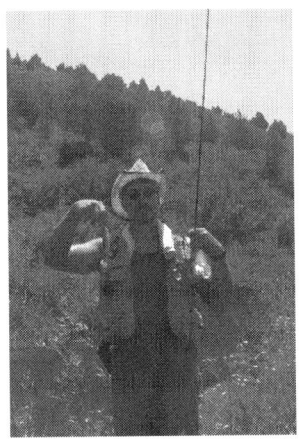

Cryotherapy

River Fishing
After Going Blind

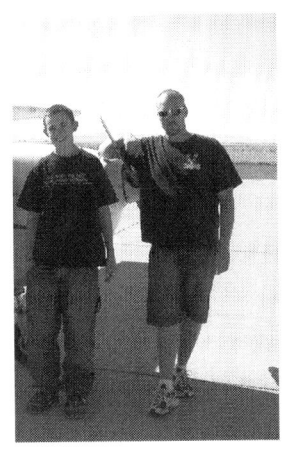

Getting Ready To Fly

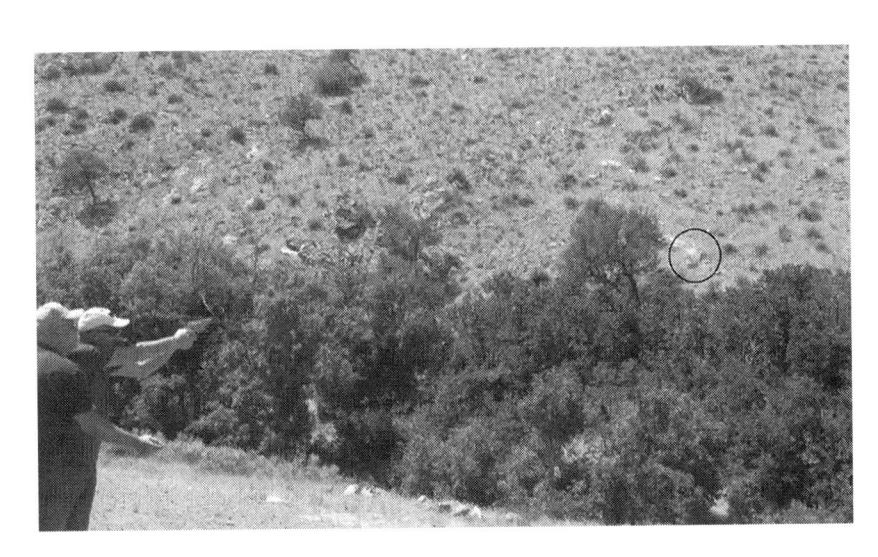

Shooting Blind

113

Part 3
The New Me

14

A New Family

"There comes a time when you have to choose between turning the page and closing the book."

— *Josh Jameson*

Cindee became pregnant at the end of our junior year. She was afraid to tell her parents, as they already had a dislike for me. In their eyes, I was one step away from Hannibal Lecter. It was her younger sister who told her parents, then they confronted us. As expected, this did not cement a good relationship between her parents and me. It was more like pouring salt onto a slug.

For several weeks after we broke the news to them, her father wouldn't even look at me and her mother had nothing nice to say about or to me. Cindee always had a great relationship with her dad, but he was hurt, and it took days for him to speak to her.

The next few months were very frustrating. Cindee and I were fighting to be together and to get married. Her parents were against us, saying that we were too young, we didn't know what love was, and that the odds were against us. We didn't care about that; we knew we were in love.

We knew that we were right for each other. We were going to make it work one way or another.

Through this period, Cindee and I started arguing, and there was a lot of tension between us. My anger had returned, and I was falling back into some of my old habits. I felt as if my world of peace and harmony was collapsing all around me.

That was when the guilt trips began. When we couldn't be together, I would tell Cindee it was because she wasn't fighting hard enough for us. At that point, I felt like I was only allowed those few short years of peace and happiness, and then the world yanked the rug out from under me, thrusting me back into the hell that I had lived for so long. Even the smallest alteration of plans would set me off, and it made everybody's conviction even stronger that we would never make it.

Still, we carried out our plans to marry. Cindee and I used one of our classes at school to design our wedding announcement, and the teacher gave us credit for it. He allowed us to make the template at school, and we took it to a printer, cutting the cost by more than half. We borrowed backdrops and centerpieces from a neighbor, trying to spend the least amount as possible. My parents had just paid for my sister's wedding and they were broke. So were we, and we had to save whatever we could for the baby.

Despite weeks of arguing, fighting and threatening, on November 14th, 1985, Cindee and I were married. It was the happiest day of my life. We were married in the church because it didn't cost anything to reserve it for the day. It was a Thursday evening and it was also the only day that month when it hadn't rained or snowed. Cindee wore a flowing white gown—the top was made of lace and appliqued flowers and was pleated from the waist down. For 1985, it was a very classy and modest gown. With the exception of watching my child's birth, when she walked out and I saw her for the first time in that dress, it was by far the single most beautiful sight I had ever seen. I believe I stopped breathing and honestly didn't care if I ever started again.

A NEW FAMILY

You know how, in the movies, everything just disappears around two people, and the world seems to stop spinning? That was me, surrounded in a whirlwind of love. Time stopped, all that moved was her and me; she appeared to just glide towards me. My life was at the climax of perfection. God had sent me an angel, and I didn't know why.

I wore a white tuxedo. I wasn't at all happy with this choice of color, but I wore it because it was what Cindee wanted. I think it's what her mom wanted, and she never says, *"No"* to her mom. Now me being the rebel as always, I had my way of mutiny. I wanted to wear a dark tuxedo, and since that wasn't happening, I decided dark socks would be.

But then I felt like dark socks wouldn't make a strong enough statement, so I found a pair of long tube socks that were striped in black, of course. Ta-Da! Mission accomplished. Bold enough to make a statement but subtle enough to not really be noticed, until…the pictures! Those stripes showed right through my white tuxedo. Yeah, I know. I'm kind of an ass, but it really could have been worse.

My wife's best friend's dad performed the ceremony. This was very important to her because she was so close to the family and it was like having her own father reciting the vows. When it came time to cut the cake, I was so careful not to make a mess, being ever so gentle when I fed the piece of cake to Cindee. She, on the other hand, made a complete mess by shoving the cake in my face, up my nose, and everywhere in between.

The rest of the evening was spent dancing, laughing, kissing, hugging and smiling—the biggest smiles any man could wear. Later that night, after all of the festivities were over, and we were completely exhausted, we dropped into bed with the agreement that we would wake early Friday morning and attend school as husband and wife. YEAH. That didn't happen.

After our wedding, we moved into the basement of my parent's home. They had spent years fixing it up to accommodate their family, and then set it up as an apartment. There were two bedrooms, a living room, bathroom, kitchen and even a washer and dryer. Living with our parents wasn't the best situation for a newly married couple, but we were in love and needed to save as much money as we could.

By this time, we were six months pregnant and everything was going well. We were learning to be a family, and preparing the best we could for it to get larger. I was working construction at the time which meant that my work was very sporadic, and the pay wasn't consistent. Little did I know that this was going to set a precedence for my income for most of my life.

For the next thirty years, Cindee and I never had another argument. We would have discussions and disagreements, and it wasn't always flowers and sunshine, but we worked together. From the smallest of worries to the biggest of disappointments, we were a team, working it out.

15

And Then There Were Four

"Build me a son, O Lord, who will be strong enough to know when he is weak, and brave enough to face himself when he is afraid, one who will be proud and unbending in honest defeat, and humble and gentle in victory."

— *Douglas MacArthur*

On the day my son was born, I was working on a job site, like any typical day. I worked six days a week, ten hours a day to make as much money as possible. My contractor's wife showed up. She told me that my wife had been taken to the hospital. I was working with several other individuals who finished the job and cleaned up for me, so I could leave immediately and go be with her.

When I arrived, I was led into a small room where my wife was waiting. She was glowing with the pending arrival, and I rushed to her side. Her water broke while she was at work. It was the first Monday in February, and at the time, she was working at the credit union branch on the local air base. That meant that it was payday for the Air Force Base—social security and retirees included—and the line was extremely long. You can imagine the looks on their faces when she announced that her water had broken, and she would be closing her window.

Many were congratulating her, but others were upset that the line would slow down. When her mom arrived to take her to the hospital, she brought her a bathrobe instead of clean clothes. Probably not the best idea, because now she wasn't just embarrassed because her water broke, but she also had to walk out in front of these insensitive, *'I want my money now'* people, wearing a bathrobe.

As they approached the exit gate on base, it was as if she was on an episode of Candid Camera (for you young people that was the original 'Punk'd'). The guards had closed the gate and they were stuck in traffic. This only lasted for a few minutes, and they made it to the hospital at about 4:00 p.m.

They were monitoring her contractions and waiting for the anesthesiologist to arrive. By the time he arrived, my wife was dilated and her contractions were very close together.

Because of this, the doctor performing the epidural was having a hard time finding the tiny sac where the medication should be injected. He tried several times without success, and we were beginning to believe that she was going to give birth without any pain relief.

I don't have a hard time watching people get shots or poked with needles; my sister is a nurse, and she would practice on me. In fact, most medical and even surgical procedures are fascinating to me. I took pictures of one of my surgeries as it was going on. The surgeon thought I was crazy to ask for a local anesthetic instead of being unconscious so that I could watch.

However, watching this doctor try to hit the epidural sac—missing—attempting again—missing again—and continuing on this way for about half an hour, made my stomach start to turn and I had to look away. When he finally found the correct location for the injection and administered the anesthesia, there was a large bruise on my wife's back and a puddle of blood on the sheets. I learned a valuable lesson that day; the one place that you never want to pass out is in a hospital. They take that shit seriously.

AND THEN THERE WERE FOUR

I wasn't allowed to participate in my sons birth. I was only allowed to stand next to my wife's head to comfort her. The doctor was older and, in his eyes, it wasn't the place of the father to be intimately involved in the birth. After six hours of labor, at 10:20 p.m., my son was brought into this world. I was so excited; words cannot explain the joy I felt. I had a son! And he was pink and perfect and his little cry was like a symphony to me. The nurses bathed him, wrapped him in a blanket and placed him in my arms.

I was surprised that they allowed me to hold him, they didn't do skin to skin contact like they do now. Back then they usually rushed the infants to be assessed and placed in an incubator, while the mother was being tended to and medically cleared. But they handed him to me and allowed me to take him to the nursery.

I held him—loved him—and cried tears of joy. Neither my wife nor I even bothered to look past his beautiful face. Back then there weren't ultrasounds or the 3-D imaging that they have now. We didn't even know the sex of our child or if there were any physical defects until after he was born. We had picked out a boy and girl name. If it was a boy, we both liked the name Curtis Ryan. But after he was born, it just didn't fit.

The nurse told me that I could take him out into the waiting area so everyone could see him. When I walked out into the hallway, our families stood and approached me. I remember hearing, *"Well, what is it?"* With tears in my eyes, I said: *"It's a Tyler."*

My mother and mother-in-law immediately started looking him over, like nervous hens with their brood of chicks. Checking for all ten fingers and toes, as well as all of the other equipment that he should have—something that never crossed my mind. I was in love with him no matter what. I just knew I had a son and to me, he was perfect.

They removed the blanket and I heard them gasp. There was a look of fear and shock on their faces. My mother-in-law immediately started to cry, and my mother just placed her hand over her mouth. *"What's wrong with his foot?"*

I looked down to see that my son had been born with a clubfoot. It didn't even faze me; it didn't change how I felt or the love that I had in my heart. He was alive, he was healthy, and he was ours.

It was customary back in 1986 to have at least an overnight stay and they usually kept you for two days after a child was born. However, the billing office at the hospital told us that, since both mom and baby were healthy, we could leave as soon as the doctor released them. The entire process was less than 24 hours, and that would save us half the cost.

We left early the following morning, about 18 hours after Tyler was born. Because of the deduction in the bill, the total was just over $900 and we paid it in full when we checked out. We made arrangements with the doctor and anesthesiologist, and for years, I teased my son that the doctor still owned the title to him.

We stayed for about a month in a small room in the basement of my in-law's home because my wife felt more comfortable there with a new child. After only one day, we had Tyler back in the hospital. He was a remarkable shade of yellow and the doctors were quite concerned.

When my wife was born, she had to have a complete blood transfusion due to jaundice, and at this point, we believed that my son would follow that tradition. We placed him in direct sunlight during the day, and under an ultraviolet light with a bandage around his eyes at night.

We had to take him to the doctor every day, sometimes twice a day, to have his blood tested, until slowly his bilirubin dropped. They had to test him so many times; his feet were covered in bruises and scabs. It is an incredibly heart-wrenching thing to watch a child that's only a couple of days old be jabbed in the bottom of his feet to get enough blood to test. And not just any child, but your child. The one you brought into existence. The child that holds onto your heart like nothing else on this planet.

When I would look into his face, I saw nothing but joy and love. To watch this, day after day, being poked and prodded and thinking of all of the other medical procedures this tiny little body would have to endure brought me to tears. And this was only the beginning of his life.

When he was two weeks old, we started seeing a specialist for his foot. We had to go in every six days to have a new cast put on to try and correct it. We were still without insurance, and we were struggling to make all of these payments to the doctors. Every cast cost $81. After about three months of casts, our pediatric orthopedist decided to cut the cost in half, because Tyler was only using a third of the plaster that a regular cast would use. For six months this continued—every six days a new cast, and every six days more pain and suffering for my child.

My father-in-law worked with a guy who was a Shriner, and he sponsored Tyler for admission to Shriner's Hospital for Crippled Children. From that day on, all of Tyler's medical treatments would be free.

I remember our first day as we approached the run-down building; we were met with the stench of disinfected mold and stale air. We entered and were put into a waiting room with several other families and children waiting to be seen.

We had no idea we would spend all day just waiting our turn. With the exception of the surgeon, we never saw the same doctor twice. The doctors were all volunteering their time, and they came from all over the world. They were some of the greatest, most loving, caring people on the planet. It amazes me to this day the work that they do with children from all over the world.

The rooms were painted with different scenes. One would have a jungle scene, another a fish scene, and so on. Once the doctors arrived, they gave total attention to my son. They made a game plan, which included surgery, to correct the bones and the tendons that had grown incorrectly, then casting again for several months, and finally braces.

When it was time for the surgery, the hospital's procedure was to keep the child overnight, and the surgery would be performed the following morning. The parents were to leave and then come back after the surgery. There were no accommodations to spend the night at the hospital. Tyler was initially scheduled for surgery at six months old, but he got sick the evening prior.

We rescheduled his surgery date for three months later, as this was the next available appointment. This time, my wife refused to leave my son's side. She insisted she would sleep on the floor rather than allow our nine month old son to go through this by himself. The hospital finally gave in and found a chair for her to sleep in. They put Tyler's crib and the chair in a room slightly bigger than a closet, so they could have a little privacy.

I drove back and forth to the hospital every day, leaving late at night and arriving before dawn. Many times I don't even remember how I made it to the hospital or back home because I was on autopilot. I will admit there were some very close calls where I almost crashed or collided with other vehicles because I was asleep behind the wheel.

I agonized as I watched my newborn son all the way through to the age of two, learning to crawl, walk and stand with the aid or hindrance of these casts and braces.

As Tyler grew, he was happy and healthy, and he laughed and played just like every other child. He didn't know that he had a disability. We never treated him like he did, either. He learned to crawl while in a brace that separated his feet and held them pointed outward. He would swing his legs back and forth like a fish tail; his little butt wiggling and twisting. We would laugh and giggle and he would laugh right along with us.

We weren't laughing at him, we were laughing because of his ingenuity and we were amazed at his accomplishment. As Tyler grew, he did everything that other children did. He could run and play and even played baseball and soccer. His life was everything we hoped it would be.

"You're not rich until you have something money can't buy."

— Garth Brooks

AND THEN THERE WERE FOUR

For anyone who has children, you understand the sheer joy that those lovely little angels can give. The love that they offer is unconditional and all they want in return is two loving arms, food and a dry butt.

There were two phrases I regularly heard as I was growing up. The first, *"He'll never live to be thirteen"*. This continued in two or three year intervals until I got married. At that point, my mom declared she was no longer financially responsible for my medical expenses and she could rest a bit easier.

The other statement that I always heard was, *"I hope you have one just like you!"* I used to believe that it was just said in frustration and that she didn't mean it. However, I have since learned that the curse is real. Of course, my mom didn't want me to have a child who was always broken or dangling on the edge of death. She was referring to my other quality; I was a smart ass and wasn't afraid to use it. I still have this quality, if you want to call it that. I prefer to say I'm honest, and most of the time, people don't want to hear the truth. To this day, it still gets me in trouble.

When my wife became pregnant with our second child, we were ecstatic. My son was still in the walking braces and had a long road to go before his feet were corrected, but we loved him so much, and we couldn't imagine anything greater than having a second child.

With my daughter, things were a lot different. When we made an appointment with the doctor, we found that things had changed quite a bit in the last year and a half. The doctor that we chose was much more progressive and a lot more fun. To give you an example, at one of our appointments, he gave my wife and me a little scare.

As he did the ultrasound, he put the transducer on one side of my wife's abdomen so that we could hear the heartbeat. He then very seriously said, *"There's one baby,"* then moved it to the other side of her abdomen and, once again, there was a heartbeat and he said, *"There's the second one."* My wife and I just stared at each other in total shock, neither one of us able to say a word. He laughed and said, *"Just kidding, there's only one."*

Several months prior to the arrival of my daughter, I had quit my construction job and gone back to school full time. I needed a better job, where I could get some insurance and a steady paycheck. I was studying electronics and was working towards an electronic engineering degree. It was a very difficult time for us. My wife was working full time, and that was our only source of income. I had received several grants and a small scholarship to go to school, so fortunately, the cost of school was negligible.

However, we had other bills and obligations. After months of living on our own, we moved back into my parent's home. This allowed us, once again, to save money, knowing that we would have more upcoming debt. We had insurance, thanks to my wife's full-time job. And even though we would struggle, it didn't matter to us. We were excited and we would make due no matter what. I was so happy knowing that we would have one more little person in our family.

In the two years since my son was born, ultrasounds had advanced dramatically. The doctor was able to see the sex of the baby. My wife had decided that she wanted to be surprised as with my son, however I didn't. After a doctor's visit, my wife left the room, and the doctor told me what he believed the sex of the baby was. My wife was so adamant about it being a secret that I promised her I would not tell her what the doctor said to me.

Later that day she decided she wanted to know and asked me to tell her. I refused, reminding her I promised I wouldn't tell her. This argument went on for several hours until I finally told her if she wanted to know she would have to contact the doctor herself. So she did.

At first, the doctor's office wouldn't tell her, because she had been so adamant about not knowing. However, after some persuasion, they told her we were having a little girl. We were beyond happy knowing that now we would have a boy and a girl.

On the day that my daughter was born, I woke up to go to school, and my wife was getting ready to go to work. My wife kept experiencing contractions, so she contacted work to let them know.

AND THEN THERE WERE FOUR

I had previously informed my professors that this day was coming, and they were all very willing to work with me.

One of my finals was scheduled for that day; it was a test that my degree would depend on. This was the type of test that, once I started it, I would have to finish or take an 'F' for the class. I asked Cindee several times if she thought I should start the test; knowing that it would be several hours before I would be able to complete it. She didn't think that she would have the baby until later that day at least, and there would be plenty of time, so I decided to take my test.

When I arrived at school and entered the classroom, the professor already had the room set up and ready to go, so I could walk right in and begin. I went into the testing cubicle and just as I was sitting down, I heard his telephone ring. I stood back up, walked back into his office and handed him my test just as he was hanging up.

Sure enough, it was Cindee, calling the school to tell me she was headed to the hospital. Fortunately, the seal had not been broken on the test so I would be allowed to retake it, due to the circumstances.

The doctor arrived, checked Cindee and informed us that we only had a couple of hours to wait. He didn't want to go back to the clinic, knowing he would be called back in such a short time, so the two of us sat just outside my wife's room and watched the current Bill Cosby special on HBO. We laughed and joked with each other while Cindee was struggling through her labor pains. It was so wrong.

There was a particular part in this special where Bill Cosby was describing childbirth. He said that Carol Burnett explained labor pains as; *"Taking your bottom lip and pulling it over your head."* The doctor and I were just howling with laughter as we were watching this. He, of course, related to it a lot more than I did. I found it funny that we were enjoying ourselves while Cindee was in the other room experiencing what Carol Burnett just described.

When it was time for my daughter to enter this world, there was a unique bond created that lasts to this day. I took my place alongside my wife as I had done with my son. I didn't realize that this was not going to be my role in the delivery of my daughter. The doctor looked at me and said: *"What are you doing up there?"* I looked at him with dumbfounded astonishment, not even really sure that's what he said. He looked at me again and said, *"Your place is down here."*

Now I love my wife dearly, and I would do anything to make her comfortable, but at that particular moment, I forgot she was even in the room. The only thing I knew was this doctor was allowing me to deliver my daughter. I would be the first person that ever touched her body and it was up to me to bring her into this world safely. The absolute wonder, joy, and pure exhilaration that I was feeling at that moment was indescribable.

I was watching this miraculous event unfold in front of me, the doctor right by my side guiding me, telling me what to do. I remember as the head started to crown, somebody in the room asked if she had hair. I was so excited I sounded like a 12 year old girl as I screamed, *"She has lots of hair!"* After the head was delivered, the doctor noticed that she was slightly blue in color, so he immediately moved me out of the way and took over. The umbilical cord was wrapped around her neck twice.

My heart was pounding so hard, and I feared there were going to be complications or problems. I remember feeling as if I couldn't breathe. The world seemed to stop for that moment in time. As the doctor unwound the cord, her color immediately returned and everything was back to normal. Once again, the doctor returned me to my place delivering my daughter.

He told me that everything was going to happen very quickly and to make sure that I held on to the baby because she was going to be slippery. Once her shoulder cleared, the rest of my baby girl was immediately delivered. I remember hearing or reading doctors describe this process as a *"Woosh,"* and believe it or not, that is the perfect description.

The doctor told me to lower the baby's head and shoulder, and before I could take my next breath, I was holding my daughter. The doctor took her from me, and they cleared her nose and throat of the mucus. She started to breathe and cry. Once again I had experienced an incredible moment in my life; I had just delivered my child. From that moment on, she knew she had me wrapped around her little finger. I can't swear to it, but I do believe she even had a little smile on her face from the realization.

16

Cops And Robbers

"Knowing your own darkness is the best method for dealing with the darkness of other people."

— *Carl Jung*

Ever since I was a small boy, I wanted to be a police officer. I know what you're thinking; *'But you were following a path where all of the people you hung around ended up in jail or prison.'* Like I said, I was never really like them.

I used the fact that I was such a *'trouble maker'* to allow my career in law enforcement to work for me. I knew when people were lying, and I could find almost anyone who tried to elude me because I used those same tactics in my younger years. My experiences came back around again to my benefit. My formal education continued with the second degree I received, which was in criminal justice and criminal psychology. However those degrees don't rival what I gained from life experiences.

Law enforcement gave me the opportunity to understand helping others. I tell people all the time that there are two types of officers;

The pretty-boys—they're the ones who got all of the girls, were on the football team, were the most popular and so on. They look exceptionally sharp in their uniforms and get a lot of phone numbers and dates rather than doing actual police work.

The nerds—they were beat up all through school, were regularly picked on and considered to be outcasts in some way. They're the ones who have something to prove; they're out there to show how big of a person they are and to fight back against everything that happened to them in school. They are extremely overactive; always stopping cars, writing citations, making arrests, using their power to the fullest extent because they have a point to prove.

I didn't fit either of these types. I wasn't a popular kid in school but not picked on either. I loved my job because of the opportunities to help others and also to prove that I could be something other than ignored.

I did have a point to prove, but in my case, I needed to show that I could be something, and it started at home rather than high school. It wasn't the jocks or the popular kids I needed to prove something to; it was my father. I needed to prove him wrong, and everybody else who said I would never amount to anything. I needed to show that I could hold my own and that I could help and be there for others.

This drove me to succeed. Eventually, I became our department's senior firearms instructor and armor. I was certified as an instructor in many other areas, as well as a certified dog handler.

One of my favorite experiences was becoming a D.A.R.E. Officer. For those who are unfamiliar with D.A.R.E., it stands for Drug Abuse Resistance Education. It's a program that was developed for elementary age children to help educate them in how to say no to drugs and alcohol.

For me, the best part of this program was that my own two children became my students. The first year that I taught, my son was in the graduating class, and the last year, my daughter was. As part of their graduation from the program, the kids write an essay on what they learned through the year. Those essays are submitted anonymously then read and judged, and the top three essays are given an award.

My daughter's essay was chosen. I was so proud to give her that award of achievement. After teaching the D.A.R.E. program for three years, I was nominated and received the D.A.R.E. officer of the year award for the state of Utah.

It's a very prestigious award among D.A.R.E. officers. Your teaching skills, knowledge and your interaction with the children are all evaluated. The officers, their chiefs, mayors, and even the governor of Utah attended this award ceremony. It was a great honor to be chosen from the hundreds of D.A.R.E. officers in the state.

My greatest achievement was being certified as a Drug Recognition Expert or D.R.E. This is a program that teaches how to recognize drugs and how they affect the human body. It's hard to get accepted into this very extensive and intensive school.

I was required to learn the different types of drugs and their symptoms, along with anatomy, medical terminology and adverse reactions. There were times that judges would call me at my house to request I appear in their courtroom to answer questions or to evaluate individuals that may be under the influence while in court.

I travelled the country to law enforcement agencies, teaching both the standardized field sobriety testing and the drug recognition expert program to police officers and military officers. I also taught a revised version of these to parents and church groups.

It always amazed me when I would bring out some of the paraphernalia; parents would say, *"My child has one of those, I thought it was just a lava lamp"*.

Corporations and companies hired me so that they were better able to evaluate the individuals who worked for them, making their work environment safer. I also assisted in helping them write drug policies for their companies.

Seeing the amount of impaired individuals and the different drugs out on the streets always amazed me. I never could wrap my head around why people chose to do this.

During my law enforcement career, I had some fascinating experiences with people on drugs. Once, I was called to a medical emergency along with paramedics and an ambulance, where we were told that a 21 year old had a seizure, fell and hit his head. Typically law enforcement is not dispatched to medical emergencies, but apparently they believed that there was something suspicious about this.

I arrived on the scene, and as I entered the house, there was a young man who weighed approximately 100 lbs laying on the floor, face up, unconscious, with blood coming from his nose and ears. I asked how long he had been unconscious, and the people in the house told me about 10 minutes.

I asked what he had taken, and everyone in the house just froze in fear. I received no answer. I explained to them that we could not help him if we didn't know what was going on. That I wasn't there to arrest them, I just needed to know what he had taken.

Finally, an individual spoke up, and I learned that he smoked some pot that day. I was then told that, after he smoked pot, he started acting crazy and passed out. When I was younger, I watched movies about exorcisms and demon possession; even then not believing what they were portraying on screen. The way bodies floated off the ground or performed unparalleled acts of strength. This day, however, I believed I was in one of those movies.

The young man's eyes opened, and he came to a standing position by pushing himself straight up off the floor with his arms. He never bent his legs or used any other body part for assistance. It was as if he slapped the floor hard enough to push his entire body into the air, still straight and rigid as a plank.

I scurried backward like a cat from water as he righted himself, screaming at me in gibberish that was reminiscent of those demons. I was doing my best to calm him down, but I wasn't even able to calm myself. I doubted my own eyes.

He became terrified and backed himself into a corner of the room. He was trying to speak to me, but all that came out was that same gibberish. I continued trying to calm him down and assure him that he would be okay, but to no avail. In his fit of panic, he picked up a stereo speaker and crushed it between his hands like a graham cracker, still screaming at me incoherently.

The entire room fled in terror leaving the two of us alone. With all of my training, and outweighing him by well over 100 pounds, I knew if he got a hold of me, I wouldn't have a chance. Whatever was coursing through his veins gave him the strength of the Hulk, even with his tiny body.

In the county I worked, the deputy sheriffs were also paramedics, which worked to my advantage in this particular incident. The two paramedics arrived on scene seconds after he crushed the stereo speaker. The splinters and shards of wood lay on the floor, and he was trampling them to dust. However, the wall of the house posed a bigger challenge than the speaker—at least for the moment.

The deputies both weighed in at well over 200 pounds. The three of us decided that the paramedics would grab him and drag him out of the corner, and I would handcuff him to protect him as well as us. As they rushed in, this young man who looked like a stick figure in comparison grabbed one of the paramedics in each hand and tossed them across the room and into the kitchen like rag dolls. I was in disbelief as they flew through the air 15 or 20 feet.

As the deputies scrambled to pick themselves back up, he tried to run for the door, and I dove at him like a linebacker. My sheer momentum knocked his small frame to the ground as I landed on top of him.

The ambulance arrived, and there were two E.M.T.'s aboard. With five people to subdue him, we only had to wrestle him for several minutes. We were finally able to get a set of handcuffs on him, but he was still out of control and screaming even louder in his demon tongue. He was pulling so hard on the handcuffs that it appeared he would break them or his arms trying to get free.

For safety, he was strapped onto a backboard and then on top of a gurney. He was trying so hard to escape from the straps that as he jerked around, he would lift the gurney off the ground in little bounces.

We later found out that his cousin had the same issue, and one of the neighboring police agencies was called to his residence as well. After several hours in the hospital, they both started to wake up, and neither of them knew what had happened or why they were in the hospital. After the blood test came back, we learned that they were both under the influence of PhenylCyclohexyl Piperidine or as most people know it—P.C.P. They had purchased some marijuana that had been laced with the drug, without them being aware of it.

Dealing with this type of drug and the effects on the people that used it, became commonplace for me as I became part of the state D.R.E. team. We would evaluate individuals under every type of drug imaginable. We were even some of the first to come in contact with several of the new drugs that are out on the street today.

Beyond those experiences, I had many enjoyable times in law enforcement as well. Once I was dispatched to an alarm at a residence. The caller said that he was unsure of what type of alarm, and I was being sent to evaluate before any further fire or medical personnel responded. It is procedure to send two officers in the event it is an intruder alarm.

I arrived, and the caller pointed me to the house where the alarm was sounding. As I walked toward the house, the second officer, Dale, pulled up. We immediately recognized the sound of a smoke detector inside the residence. As we looked around, we could see smoke coming out of the swamp cooler that was mounted on the roof of the house. I informed dispatch to send fire and paramedics to my location.

We searched the entire residence for an open door or window, with no luck. I made the decision to kick in the front door to determine if anybody was inside the home. I kicked the front door with enough force to send it completely off the hinges. It flew into the house approximately 10 feet and landed on the stairs that led to the upper living portion of the home.

We entered and immediately were hit by thick plumes of smoke, as it rolled out of the open door. We crouched down to avoid the smoke as much as possible and started searching the home. In the living room, I found a female on the couch; she was unconscious but breathing. We also noticed a significant amount of smoke and flames coming from the kitchen area in the home.

I grabbed the woman and threw her over my shoulder, carrying her out of the burning home. Dale went into the kitchen to try to extinguish the fire as much as possible but realized it was too much. He left the kitchen to search the home for other residents.

He found an unconscious male in the bedroom. He regained consciousness as Dale attempted to pick him up. He was trying to escort the man out of the house, but in his daze, the man tried to turn off the stereo and straighten up the home; he didn't understand what was going on.

Dale was finally able to escort him out of the home and onto the front lawn, where he sat next to the woman I had carried out. I reentered and, after finding no other occupants in the home, I exited the structure only to find that the male owner of the home had gone back in and Dale had to retrieve him a second time.

We learned from the occupants that they had come home late from a day at the lake and started to cook something to eat. Being exhausted from a day in the sun, they both fell asleep. The pan, food and cupboards above the stove had all caught fire while they slept. The amount of smoke and carbon monoxide combined with the exhaustion had rendered them both unconscious and delirious, so neither of them heard the smoke detector going off.

As the paramedics and ambulance arrived on scene, the female went into respiratory arrest. They loaded both occupants and headed to the nearest hospital. I didn't realize it before because of the excitement, but I was having difficulty breathing. My lungs were on fire, and I was beginning to become light headed. I stripped off my shirt and Kevlar vest so that I could breathe better. A second set of paramedics arrived with the fire department, and Dale and I were transported to the hospital and treated for smoke inhalation.

Two months later, Dale and I were invited to their wedding, where they thanked us for saving their lives and allowing them the opportunity to see this day.

Sadly, after ten years in law enforcement, I realized that I did not fit the *'cop'* profile. With a dislike for donuts and coffee and a unique ability to make people laugh while dealing with the public, I was soon outcast by my peers. Even after all this time, I still seemed to be longing for that feeling of belonging and satisfaction.

17
It's All Downhill From Here

"I have been bent and broken but—I hope—into a better shape."

— *Charles Dickens*

When I was nine years old, my dad and I, along with my uncle and cousin, were bird hunting in the west desert area of Utah. We had hiked for hours that day and never saw a single bird. As we trudged up one of the mountains, I heard a strange sound coming from the sagebrush. My father was going deaf and he had lost about 50 percent of his hearing by this stage, and it was near impossible for him to notice a lot of things.

One of those things was the sound coming from the brush. I never hunted for these birds before and had no idea what they sounded like. I tried to explain it to him; a very weird clicking sound, something I had never heard before. He dropped back a few steps, raised his shotgun up to his shoulder to be prepared for whatever came out, and instructed me to, *"Kick the bush."* I did as he said and kicked the brush several times. Nothing came out. The noise just got louder.

After attempting for several minutes to get whatever it was out, I decided maybe what I needed to do was look and see what was making the noise. I started separating the branches of the sagebrush to get a better look inside and suddenly realized I could see a small object—rattling. Utah is full of rattlesnakes but even with as much hunting, fishing and camping as I had done in my short life, this was my first encounter.

Simultaneously, I noticed the rattlesnake and it noticed me. Then it struck! The snake's fangs sank deep, and I tried to pull away, but was held for a moment by the snake. Luckily, this particular day I was wearing a pair of my father's hiking boots with three pairs of socks, so that my feet would kind of fit. The boots were extremely loose, especially around my ankles and calves. Who knew that my saving grace would be the fact that my parents couldn't afford to buy me a pair of boots that fit? The snake was attached to the loose part of the boot, avoiding contact with me completely.

It scared me so badly that I turned and ran down the hill about 50 yards before stopping. My father, still standing in the same place, stared at me dumbfounded. He did not understand what just happened, and what I was yelling at him.

Now my father can curse and swear right along with the best of them, but me being only nine years old, I wasn't supposed to. What I thought I said was, *"It's a snake"* What came out was, *"IT'S A FUCKING SNAKE!"* Luckily for me, his hearing loss prevented him from completely understanding what I said.

Reluctantly, I trudged back up the hill to my father, and there was that rattle louder than ever, still in the sagebrush. When I got close enough to my dad, I yelled at him, *"It's a snake."* I remembered my language this time. He didn't believe me at first, repeatedly asking if I was positive? I tried to figure out where I went wrong with my very specific statement.

After what seemed like an eternity, but was probably about 30 seconds, he decided he would look for himself. He was a little smarter and less brave about it than I was. The difference being that I didn't know what I was looking at, but he did. And he was armed. He used the barrel of the shotgun to move the branches of the sagebrush apart so that he could look down inside. As I stood there and watched him, it was as if the devil himself had jumped out of that bush.

The shotgun went off as my dad's finger instinctively pulled the trigger. It was a surprise to all three of us. He told me that all he saw was the rattle, and the gun went off; he didn't even remember pulling the trigger. Unfortunately, I could still hear it rattling just fine. It was still alive in there. He once again used the barrel of the shotgun to move away the branches until he could see the snake's head. The gun roared, and the rattle stopped.

The first shot hit the snake in the middle of its body—it didn't kill it, but it couldn't crawl away either. As it was attempting to get away, it could only slither to the point where it was shot, and then it stopped, allowing my dad to deliver the fatal shot. We retrieved the snake from under the bush. It was approximately three and a half feet long and had seven buttons on the rattle.

I still have that rattle, to remind me to be careful and always pay attention to my surroundings. I also kept the boots I was wearing that day for a long time, to point out the fang marks.

Once my son and I started hunting together, he became my safety system. He was always the one who came to save me from one disaster after another. He was there to lift me back up or pull me back down, whichever was necessary.

We still talk and laugh today about two of the most frightening times. The first one was we were goose hunting near the Great Salt Lake, where there are salt flats between the marshes and the lake. We hiked out through the marshes, across the salt flats, and into the second set of wetlands. Just like all of the times before, the geese flew right over us, unaware that we were even there.

As they came over, we both fired, and several geese fell from the flock. One of them flew across one of the marshes and onto the salt flats on the other side. My dog was retrieving the birds which had fallen closest and didn't see that bird go down. I knew that I couldn't just leave it there and wait for the dog, so I told my son that I would go after it, and if I couldn't catch it I'd have him bring the dog to me.

I walked down the dike which separated the marsh from the salt flats, until I found a spot that appeared to be relatively shallow and narrow enough that I could wade across it to get to the flats on the other side. As I started across, I realized I had found a spot where the mud underneath the water was deeper than I was tall.

The mud in this area of the marsh is very much like quicksand; sometimes it just continues to go down deeper and deeper. There are tales of jets from the Air Force Base that have crashed into the Great Salt Lake and have never been recovered. Even with the military's high-tech sonar and ground penetrating radar, the planes are buried so deep from their high-speed impact that they just disappear.

I had started to cross the swamp, when I came upon one of these areas. I immediately began to sink and the more I struggled, the deeper I sank until I was literally up to my armpits in water. I was holding my arms above my head, realizing that I needed to stop struggling. Panic set in, and I started to fear for my life. My shotgun was on the dike, so I couldn't use it to signal for help. I had no other way to get back to dry land and I was still sinking.

I hollered for my son as loud as I could, expecting him to come running to find me; but he thought I was hollering because more geese were coming. He felt he needed to get down behind the blind so they wouldn't spook. I hollered for him again and, at that point, he heard the panic in my voice. He stood up and looked for me, but he couldn't see me anywhere. He felt a rush of fear go over him because he, too, knew what the marsh was like.

He started running down the dike and, in his panic, ran right past me. The water was creeping up to my neck at this point, and I screeched out, *"Tyler!"* as he ran by. He stopped and looked around for a few seconds, not realizing I was right in front of him, sinking.

He finally saw me and he picked up my shotgun, unloaded it, and reached out until I could grab onto the barrel. He then pulled against that mud until I finally broke free and he was able to pull me all the way up onto the dike. We recovered all of our geese that day, and I lived. But that fear never left me. There are still times I wake up in a cold sweat and panic, dreaming about that experience. I have never hunted the marshes by myself since.

The second experience was a time we were in the Uinta Mountains in northeastern Utah, and we were hunting deer in about three feet of snow.

We set out opening morning and hiked to a spot where we had seen deer, and that I believed would be a good pass-through because of the snow. I was correct. As my son and I were standing there talking, a beautiful buck walked right past us. By the time I saw it, it had already gone back into the trees, and we were unable to take a shot. We hiked around and found where it had been laying. We left the area, making plans to come back that evening because there was a good chance he'd return.

We returned that night, but we never saw the deer. I knew that since we were hunting in the snow, we needed to start back to camp earlier than usual. We began making our way about an hour before sunset, hiking and talking, looking at the beautiful scenery covered in snow. It started to get dark, and I knew the camp was still about a half hour away. I decided that we should get to the road and follow it into camp, because if anyone came looking for us, they would find us easier and faster.

As I turned to start my way down toward the road, my feet slipped on ice. They came right out from under me, and I fell straight onto my back. As I hit the ground, my head collided with a large rock that was buried under the snow, and I was knocked unconscious. I tumbled head over heels to the bottom of the mountain. Just like you see in the movies, my limp body flipping and twisting as momentum increased. I finally stopped where the slope and the roadway met.

My son did his best to try to catch up to me to keep me from rolling down the hill, but the snow and ice slowed him down. When he finally reached me at the bottom of the hill, I was just returning to consciousness. It was like waking up from a dream, not knowing what was real and what wasn't. It appeared to be bright daylight, although I knew it was supposed to be dark. I thought to myself,

IT'S ALL DOWNHILL FROM HERE

How long have I been lying here?
Have I been here all night?

I knew that couldn't be true, but I couldn't figure out anything else. I was suffering from what is called aphasia; my mind couldn't make sense of anything. It also causes an inability to understand or express speech, because of brain damage. When my son finally reached me, he knelt down, his face flushed and breathing hard. Then just as clear as can be, said…

"Mama eats turtles in the orchard!"
He actually said, *"Dad, are you okay?"* but the aphasia mixed up all his words.

I stared at him like he asked me to kill puppies, and I asked, *"What the hell did you just say?"* and what he heard was,
"A bat goes pancakes in a Buick."
Now the look of confusion on my face was mirrored by his.

He asked, *"What?"* and I heard, *"Dongle?"*
I replied, *"What?"* and he heard *"Jammy?"*

I started to realize that everything was going gray and fuzzy, then I heard the first thing I comprehended in this exchange, *"Oh shit!"* My son rolled me over to my side, and I threw up.

I have had years of medical training, and I knew what this meant; I had a brain injury. I understand now that, when it's you that has the brain damage, you do realize it, however, you still think everything is fine. As I lay there, now starting to comprehend the severity of my injuries, I realized that I couldn't stand, was having difficulty breathing and, of course, my head was throbbing.

The one thing that still stood out in my mind was, *'I can't let this show.'* My dad had beaten the idea into me that no matter what, I was never to show weakness. I should brush it off; act tough. And that's exactly what I did. I was trying to stand, and my son was holding me still to prevent further injuries. He knew he had to keep me stable and keep me talking. We had two-way radios, and he was attempting to contact our camp over and over, with no reply.

After what seemed like an eternity, but was probably only several minutes, he looked down at me and said, *"You have to move!"* I realized at this point the extent of my injuries as the initial shock and adrenalin wore off. *"I can't move!"* was the only thought I had. He reiterated, *"Dad you have to..."* before he could finish his sentence and I could retort, he reached his arms around me and, with all of his strength, stood me up.

We both fell backward into the snowbank as a pickup truck flew by us at about 50 miles an hour. The vehicle never even slowed down; it just sped by. Had I still been laying in the roadway, I would have been a casualty of that vehicle as well.

I finally got up enough strength to stand. It was extremely painful, and I was dizzy and nauseated. As we were standing there, the darkness of the night engulfing us, a second vehicle pulled up and stopped. They asked if everything was okay, and in my confusion and not wanting anyone to see me in pain or suffering, I told them we were fine, *"Just waiting for our ride to pick us up."* I told them.

My son just looked at me like I was trying to herd chickens. But still I was adamant that I was fine and that we had a ride coming. Later when my son and I discussed this, I didn't even remember the conversation or a vehicle that stopped.

My son was in a panic as to how he was going to get us off this mountain. I was starting to gain more of my senses and realized that the only option we had, was for him to leave me there and get closer to camp where the radios would make contact. After he got some help, he could then come back and get me. He argued that he did not want to leave me there. I told him it was our only chance; he needed to get back and get help.

Just as he was preparing to leave, the radio keyed, and my father-in-law's voice came over. He was at camp and was worried that we hadn't made it back. By some miracle, he got through. We had tried unsuccessfully for 20 minutes to make contact with the camp, and he had somehow gotten through. My son told him that I had fallen and was in a bad way, and that he needed to come and get us. His reply, *"I know right where you are, I'll be right there."*

I don't know how he knew where we were, but he drove right to us. He picked us up and took us back to camp. My decision to get to a road instead of going directly to camp paid off. My father-in-law tried to get me to go straight to the hospital but, of course, I couldn't let that happen.

The next morning my son drove me off the mountain to a hospital. My wife escorted me into the ER and after the nurse heard the reason for my visit, she called for the doctor to meet me in the waiting area. She was worried about my breathing and scolded me for not coming down the night before when the accident happened.

I sustained a deflated lung, three broken ribs, a cracked and bruised hip, and a major concussion. Based on that, the doctor said I should have been transported by helicopter. It took several months of recovery before I could walk without a limp and breathe without pain. My cognitive abilities would come and go, and I had a few minor side effects from the concussion. But after a while, I was back to normal…well, my normal.

I have come to realize that hunting, although a great stress reliever for me, is where I suffer most of my injuries and near death experiences. Another time I was hunting for grouse and chucker with my friend, Chris. We saw a flock of chucker scurry up a hill, and we worked our way around to flank them. As we got to the top of the hill and started down, we were confronted by a large bull moose.

The moose was just standing there, eating grass, not a care in the world. We threw some rocks toward the moose and even tried firing a shot over its head to scare it off, but the moose didn't budge. We stood and waited for about 10 minutes before he finally decided to walk off into the trees. I thought we were safe, and we started down the hillside once again.

As we walked, I heard the moose grunt and begin to charge. I turned to see him exiting the trees running right towards me at full speed. He had his antlers down like the shovel of a bulldozer. I instinctively turned and fired; I was only carrying a shotgun which is no match for a full grown bull moose. I knew it wouldn't stop him, but I thought maybe it would deter him or scare him off.

The moose never skipped a beat or a step. Before I could fire a second shot, it had run me over and pushed me to the ground. Just to give a better understanding of what it was like; the male moose have antlers that can be 60 inches in width and weigh up to 50 pounds. Average weight range of a mature Shira's moose is 600 to 1400 pounds. This one was close to the 1000 pound range.

As I lay on the ground, looking up at the underside of this moose, it appeared closer to the size of a dump truck. I once again instinctively fired my shotgun just alongside its head, hoping to scare it off. The moose started to stomp the ground with his two front legs, trying to crush me under its weight.

I somehow was able to roll my body back and forth and avoid each of the heavy blows. This Bull Moose was determined, and if either of those front hooves would have made contact with me, it would have crushed me like a bug on the sidewalk. I could feel the weight of him as each hoof smashed into the ground on either side of me, like little explosions. Dirt and rubble covered my body.

I had one shot left, and I knew the moose was not to be deterred. I brought the gun right up underneath him pressing the barrel right against its body and pulled the trigger…

I saw a giant ball of flame, and I heard the moose grunt. I thought my gun had exploded, and I believed my only option was to swing my gun like a club to defend myself. Before I could do anything, it turned and ran off down the hill away from me.

I was frightened and completely depleted of energy. I just laid my head back and closed my eyes, trying to reign in my thoughts. As I lay there with my eyes closed, I heard Chris come running up to me. He had to skirt a large stand of thick brush to get to where I was. By the time he arrived, the moose had already run off down the hill.

Exhausted, I stayed there for a few more seconds, trying to regain my composure, when I heard Chris say, *"How am I going to tell your wife that you're dead?"* I immediately opened my eyes and exclaimed, *"Oh my god, I'm dead?"* He jumped about a foot into the air and scrambled to get away from me, believing a dead man had just spoken to him.

Thinking that I was severely injured, and covered in blood, he tried to keep calm. I didn't believe that I was hurt because I couldn't find any injuries or places where I was bleeding. We finally realized that it was the blood from the moose. I don't know how, but miraculously, I escaped without injury. We attempted to locate the moose several times throughout that day to verify its injuries, but to no avail.

I have learned that the expression of *'he will never live past 13'* has extended throughout my entire life. And although my mom no longer has the burden of caretaking, she, along with everyone that knows me, still wonders what will happen next. I have had great experiences and triumphs but the things that stand out and have impacted me most are the ones that almost ended my life.

I didn't intentionally try to place myself in harms way, but it wouldn't have been as fun or memorable otherwise.

18

Make Me Laugh

"Rhetoric does not get you anywhere, because Hitler and Mussolini are just as good at rhetoric. But if you can bring these people down with comedy, they stand no chance."

—*Mel Brooks*

I started performing standup comedy as a way to express my comedic side. There was something about hearing the laughter and receiving instant gratification that began filling my emotional well. Eventually, I quit law enforcement and bought several comedy clubs.

This is what I felt I was put on this earth to do. Humor has always been one of those things that just seemed to come naturally. As long as I can remember, I've been performing. From plays at school and being the class clown, to entertaining at family parties and gatherings. I pursued this adventure into my adulthood in much the same fashion.

I learned very quickly that there is a vast difference between being funny and telling jokes. Being funny and just acting silly is ideal for family parties and gatherings. Jokes are written in a very

MAKE ME LAUGH

particular format, and they must meet certain requirements for the mind to react with laughter.

Out of everything with my dad, the best thing he did was help build my sense of humor and ability to tell stories. Throughout my life, I have been bombarded with nonsensical facts and stories that I was led to believe. My dad enjoyed gathering the young children around him and spinning a yarn or two. Many times my friends and I would be mesmerized by his stories. He would tell us about the old days, when everything was still in black and white because there was no such thing as color. It wasn't *film* that was devoid of color. It was the *world*.

"*Oh! The joy that everyone experienced when they saw color for the first time!*" he would say. And my friends believed him. How were we to know? We weren't there to see it for ourselves. My life as a child was filled with letdown after letdown as I would relay this new information to people who had no idea that this was how things were. Not to mention the trouble I'd get into as a five year old, arguing with my teacher.

The amount of testing and analyzing which took place my kindergarten year just to determine if I had some psychological issue that needed treatment was lengthy. I was proud to relay the nursery rhymes that I diligently practiced to recite the 'correct' way from my father. Imagine the shock and horror on my kindergarten teacher's face when I stood in front of the class and recited…

"*Mary, Mary quite contrary how does your garden grow? With silver bells and cockle shells and all them damn dirty ol' weeds.*"

"*Hickory Dickory Dock, the mouse ran up the clock, the clock struck one, and down he runs, and the cat gobbled him up.*"

"*Little Miss Muffet, sat on her tuffet, eating her curds and whey, along came a spider, and sat down beside her, and she took her thumb and squished it all over the place.*"

"Jack and Jill went up a hill to fetch a pail of water, Jack fell down and broke his crown, and Jill laughed her ass off."

As an impressionable young child, they made perfect sense to me. Why wouldn't a garden in a nursery rhyme have weeds? Many a summer's day was spent being punished for some wrongdoing by pulling weeds. Cats notoriously ate mice. I guarantee that there isn't a single one of you who wouldn't laugh if your friend fell down and hurt themselves. How was I to know that this was not the way the nursery rhymes went, when I was raised with things like this being said to me on a daily basis?

Imagine my mother's shock when she was called into the principal's office to discuss the possibility of her son having some mental disorder. To find out that the school psychologist had been called in to evaluate me and my psychotic delusions, to determine a course of action. And further, add the embarrassment of her having to explain that it was all my father's fault. That he had taught me those nursery rhymes as well as the other stories that I had relayed to the class.

As fallout from my childhood, I also developed an exaggerated point of view. I would entertain my kids and their friends for hours with story after story that were all fabrications from my vast imagination. My children soon learned not to ask me what something was because I would tell them in no uncertain terms what I believed it would be.

The phrase *"I'll just ask Mom."* Became commonplace, and was accompanied with disgust and cynicism from my children. Later in their lives, when they would call with a question or a problem; whenever they heard my voice, their immediate response was, *"Let me talk to Mom."*

I have since realized that this does not just apply to children or youth. It is human nature to want to believe what we are told. Many times in comedy clubs, the comedian on stage will have to remind the audience that these are *"jokes"* and not to be taken seriously.

The humorous side of me just doesn't deal well with some of the questions posed, and it is in my nature to point out how stupid they are. We have all heard the phrase "There is no such thing as a stupid question." However, I believe that certain people would be better off *not* asking questions.

Sometimes I want to respond with, *"Are you serious?"* to questions like *"How do Mexican people understand each other?"* Apparently the woman asking this question said that all she heard when they spoke was *"Bla-Bla-Bla"*.

So she wondered if Spanish speaking people heard *"Bla-Bla-Bla"* also? I explained to her that when Spanish-speaking people talk, they hear *"Bla-Bla-Bla"* and then in their head it translates into English. They think their response in English and then turn it back to *"Bla-Bla-Bla"* as they speak. She was so impressed at how fast their brain could translate and respond, when she has such a hard time with just English. The only thing I wanted to say was, *"breathe."*

I was once asked if I was a member of the military. I responded, *"No. Why?"* He said, *"Well, you just look like you're in the military."* Now at this point, common sense suggests that we should let that be the end of the conversation and just move on, all happy. However, I never have been accused of having common sense, so I promptly asked, *"So were you in those Special Ed classes in school?"* It was something about the way he looked.

The first time I performed comedy was at a family Christmas party. My mom talked me into trying my comedy in front of the family. I wrote about an hour of material, knowing I would be in front of people who would probably both encourage me and love it more than anyone, but would also be my biggest critics.

I remember the laughter coming from my family as I recited all of the jokes that I had spent hours perfecting. A brother-in-law compared me to one of his favorite comedians, stating that he hadn't laughed that hard in a long time. After this, I would practice thoughts and premises on my friends and coworkers to see what kind of reaction I would get. Their laughter became addictive—pumping through my body, exhilarating and filling me up—and I couldn't stop.

After a couple of months, my little sister, Sherry, told me she had signed me up for an open mic night in a local comedy club and that she had invited the entire family and some of our closest friends to be there.

Open mic is where experienced comedians practice fresh material and new comedians get their first chance to be on stage. I was beyond nervous; in fact, I was more frightened than I had ever felt before. I wanted this so badly that it was the only thing I could think of, and yet, I was so afraid of failure that I almost didn't go.

When I arrived, the stage manager told me I would have five minutes; the material would have to be my own and that it needed to be clean. I stood there in the club that evening listening to the comedians on stage, and I remember thinking, *"There's no way I can do this. I can't follow these people."*

I was doing everything I could to talk myself out of this thing that had consumed me for the past four months. My fear grew, my heart was pounding, I was sweating, and all I could think was that I was going to make a fool of myself.

I was introduced and stepped on stage for the first time. The bright lights hit me in the face, and the sound of my voice was echoing in the speakers. I suddenly heard the laughter of the crowd and my addiction grew. I don't believe there is a drug out there that could be this powerful. I finished my five minutes and, to be honest, I cannot remember what I even said. It felt like I had only been onstage for a few seconds. It was as if I was in a trance.

After the show, I was congratulated by the seasoned comics and even some of the audience members. The owner of the club approached me and invited me back the next week. I was on cloud nine. I don't think my feet touched the ground as I floated from the elation of accomplishment and being invited back to do it again.

I was taken under the wings of several more seasoned and professional comics. They taught me how to be a better stand-up comedian. The owner of the club took me on road trips with him.

He helped me with syntax and stage presence. I worked hard and spent as much time as I could on stage, getting as much experience as possible. After six short months, the owner signed me up for my first comedy competition.

There were 12 comedians, including myself, in the contest. The other 11 had between 10 and 15 years of experience. This would be similar to a Little League Baseball Team attempting to compete with the New York Yankees. I knew that I didn't have a chance. It was ridiculous for me to even *try* to be a part of the group of individuals that were in this competition. However, I knew that it would be one of the greatest learning experiences of my life. I expected to place last. That didn't matter to me. What mattered was that the club owner saw something in me and believed it was worth cultivating.

The competition went on for three weeks, and it covered four states. Each night, for the first round, all of the comedians would do five minutes, and the audience was allowed to vote. The top five were brought on stage for recognition, and the winning comic of that evening would do another 10 to 15 minutes.

Now, realizing that this was just a learning experience and that I had no actual chance of winning any of the nights, it was still an incredibly frightening concept for me. I only had a total of 10 minutes of material.

During the second round of the competition, our time was raised from five to ten minutes. I was really surprised I made it that far. But I would take anything that I could get and learn as much as I could.

On one of the nights, the comedians were sure that I would take 1st place. For whatever reason, the audience connected with me and my set went very well. I was especially scared and nervous, because I had used all of the material in my set. That particular night I took 3rd place. I was relieved and, at the same time, overwhelmed. Beyond thrilled I had placed against such great competition.

At the very end of the competition, the comics assured me, once again, that I would place. I felt it was one of the best sets that I had done in the entire competition. I didn't even place in the top five that night. Well, apparently coming from a law enforcement career to comedy had a few drawbacks; one of them being that a judge in the audience that night just happened to be an individual whom I had arrested years before. This person swayed the other judges, and I ended up with the lowest score of the night. (I didn't learn this until years later, after talking to the creator of the competition.)

But I wasn't discouraged. I was proud of my accomplishments to this point. I had made it to the final round and when all the tallies were added up, I took 6th place. I had gone into a situation where I knew I couldn't win, and my only desire was to come out better than when I went in. What I learned in those few weeks was more than I could have learned in a year of traveling the circuit and watching other shows. I met some of the most fantastic, genuine people. I also met some of the most cynical, jaded, and downright bitter people.

I have had the great pleasure of meeting and working with some of the biggest comedians of all time, some of whom I adored as a child and, in most cases, they turned out to be the exact type of person I hoped they were. I used to watch Louie Anderson, Sinbad, and Bobcat Goldthwait, and now I can say I've worked with them. I've also worked with Kevin Nealon, Louis CK, Greg Behrent and Harland Williams. They are some of the most genuine, kind, and caring individuals I have ever met. Also, they are hysterically funny.

I always seemed to gravitate toward comics who worked clean and were family oriented. They were and are inspirations to me. I felt like, if they could get through their family lives and come out smiling and laughing, then I could, too.

One of my favorites is Louie Anderson. You may remember him from his television cartoon series *'Life with Louie.'* I bonded with that cartoon so much because it was about his struggles with his family life and it was at a time in my life when I had just started to get over my family conflicts. When I finally got to meet Louie, I found him to be genuine, smart, funny and one of the most caring people I've ever met.

However, there were several comedians I watched and had the opportunity to work with who didn't turn out to be the type of person I expected. It was such a disappointment to find out how sarcastic and cynical they had become.

After two years of stand-up comedy, I purchased three clubs. I booked professional comedians as well as local talent. Being the owner, it allowed me to have as much stage time as I wanted. It also gave me a unique chance to sit down with all of the comics as they came through, and have writing sessions.

While booking my clubs, I had the breakthrough opportunity of my life: I hired a hypnotist. Watching his show, I was mesmerized and entertained like never before and I knew that this was what I was meant to do with my life. It hit me like a freight train; that visceral understanding that you cannot explain, you just know that it is meant to be.

I talked it over with the comedian who gave me my start and guided and cultivated me throughout the years. He had been performing stand-up for many years and is still one of the funniest people I know. He had worked in every facet of the comedy business, and his advice was always worth asking.

I enrolled in a class and learned the basics, receiving a certificate to hypnotize and my new life and career took off. For the past 15 years, it has been a rollercoaster of great and amazing things. I have performed in Las Vegas in front of 3000 people and for major corporations like Microsoft, A.O.L. Time Warner, Fox Broadcasting, and many more. From this, I have built and developed several different shows, and what's called in the business, *'Bits'*.

Now having been trained as a comedian, I had worked the comedy circuit and paid my dues. I learned from some of the very best and tried hard to make it in the business. However, I finally came to the realization that there were millions of comics trying to *'make it'* in the business, and I was just one drop in that ocean. But hypnosis? That was different. I had fallen in love with it and knew it was my way to succeed.

At the third show I ever performed, I was approached by a talent agent who was booking shows for a large comedy club. She told me that she had been in Las Vegas and California looking at hypnotists to hire for their club, and she had not seen anything as good as my show. Before even stepping foot on stage, I spent months creating and developing a show that I thought would stand out and be better than other hypnotists.

As a side note, I cannot count the number of times I have had a competitor come to my show just to steal my 'Bits' for their use. I have even had them tell me this, as if it's what we all do—steal other hypnotist's acts, as long as they're funny.

I worked very hard to perfect my show and give audiences the most fun I could create. When I lost my vision I believed it was over and my show was a thing of the past. This was very hard for me because of how much I needed my show and what it had done for me in terms of self-esteem and accomplishment.

My disability, as I explained, is very rare and unknown, and for some inexplicable reason I can see the colors fluorescent orange and fluorescent pink. Not just orange and pink; it needs to be that neon fluorescing construction sign orange. To quote a great comic and good friend of mine, Bengt Washburn…

"That bright scar your corneas orange. The orange that would give your chameleon an aneurysm."

That orange stands out like a glow stick in the dark. I can see road construction signs from about a mile away if they have the sun hitting them. I cannot read what's on them, but I know they're there. I tell people all the time I can drive. There's so much road construction all I have to do is follow the orange barrels and signs.

This is my saving grace for everything that I do. When I perform, people who come to see my shows have little to no idea that I have a vision or hearing loss. I line the stage, chairs, tables and any other obstacles that may be in the area with bright orange duct tape. I also have the club where I'm working use specially made wristbands, like the ones used for concerts, as proof of admission for the show.

The fluorescent orange and pink glow and I can follow the crowd and the participants on stage like the robot Wall-E follows the lines on the floor. Everyone believes the tape is for safety reasons. And in a way, it is, because falling off the stage is not safe.

I can perform without anyone being the wiser. I get asked all the time how I know when someone stands up or moves. How do I know when they want to high-five me and if I can't see them, how do I make contact with their hand? It's simple. *"WRISTBANDS"* I just look for the orange dot floating in the air and know that their hand is directly in front of it.

Sometimes I miss a high-five or handshake, or even the occasional person altogether. In these cases, usually the wristband is covered or they're using the opposite hand. I also have stage help that monitors the show to catch people who may fall or to assist me in things I miss, just to keep it as safe as possible.

The owner of the club where I work most often is the same man who gave me my start all those years ago. When I contacted him and told him I would like to attempt to continue working, he allowed me unlimited access to the club during the week when there weren't any shows. I was able to try different ideas of how I could continue.

After several months of taping areas of the room and stage, adjusting the lights so that it created the best ambiance as well as allowing me to still see the tape and rehearsing for numerous hours, I am still performing and the accomplishment and self-esteem are better than ever.

19

IT WASN'T ME

"I never knew how strong I was until I had to forgive someone who wasn't sorry and accept an apology I never received."

— *Unknown*

By the time I was in my mid-30's, my father was at the height of his mental illness, but still hadn't been diagnosed. Our relationship wasn't the greatest, and I had a hard time being around him. We communicated in short sentences and I always felt apprehensive. By this time, our roles had reversed. He wanted to look better in my eyes, trying to fit in and gain acceptance from me.

He also made up stories to validate things that he wanted us to believe. For instance, he would come down and talk to me about a new rifle or cartridge that was on the market and how he had met somebody—never any particular person or name—just someone that knew *so much* about that specific topic and had told him all about it.

Then, he would give me a magazine article referring to that same rifle cartridge, and all of the information that he had relayed to me—supposedly from this very informative individual—would be in that article. As I would look at the report, he would proceed to tell me that he had found the article after he talked to whomever, and it corroborated that person's statements.

My father also continued to blame everybody else but himself for all of the problems or mishaps in his life. Something would turn up missing that he had misplaced, or something would break or go wrong, and he would fault someone else.

Thus, after I was married, I spent the majority of my time with my father-in-law. He was an extremely knowledgeable mechanic, as well as a great father and mentor. He taught me more things in my first few years of marriage than I had learned in my entire life. When it came to mechanics and how to work hard for something that I wanted, he showed me by example and by assisting me, never berating me for not knowing.

He couldn't understand why I spent so much time with him, doing things at his house, and not with my own father. One summer, both my father and father-in-law were re-roofing their houses. My father-in-law wondered why I was over there helping him when I should have been helping my dad. This occurred many times, and my father-in-law asked me why I would not help my father. He always tried to push me to help him and never understood why I chose to stay away.

When my children were young, we would go with my wife's family to Yellowstone for ten days every summer. One particular year, just before we left, my father was spending time over at my in-laws. My father-in-law had a very large shop area, and my dad decided he needed to rebuild an engine and asked to borrow the space.

At first, my father-in-law tried to supervise and help him as much as he could, but he was starting to realize what type of a person my father was and how it was tough to give him advice, because he was always right.

As my father was completing his engine, he lost a bolt and couldn't find it. My father-in-law insisted that he needed to disassemble the motor to make sure that it wasn't lost somewhere in the engine. But my father argued with him that there was no way he lost that bolt in the engine. It was evident to him that one of the grandkids had taken it.

Shortly after, we left to spend ten blissful days in Yellowstone fishing, hiking and exploring. When we returned home, my father was still out in the shop. I could tell that he was angry. He was talking to himself, cursing and throwing things around. My father-in-law and I walked out to see what was going on, and he immediately started to explain how my children had ruined his engine.

He showed us a pan that had been filled with gravel and sand that he claimed he dumped out of his engine. He proceeded to tell us that one of my children had put it in there as he was rebuilding it, causing the engine to be damaged beyond repair.

He said that, as he tried to turn the engine over, it locked up because of all the sand and rocks. My father-in-law, knowing that my kids were with us in Yellowstone during the supposed sabotage, started to disassemble the motor and found the missing bolt lodged in one of the cylinders. I believe it was at that moment he realized why I spent so much time with him and refused to help my father with anything.

One night, my dad called me and asked if he could talk to me at my house. When he arrived, he was very solemn and serious. He brought with him some paperwork that I could tell he was going to use to help formulate his argument. I could tell there was something on his mind and that it was going to be somebody else's fault…and I knew that no matter what I had to say, he was going to be right.

We went down into my basement where I have a room and talked. This is when I received one of the greatest shocks of my life and realized just how far my father was willing to go to make sure he did not get blamed for anything.

He proceeded to tell me how he believed that I was not his son; that my mother had an affair with one of his friends and my three younger sisters and I were this other man's children. He explained that, because my blood type and his blood type did not match, there's no way I could be his son. Another of his reasons was that he was only 5'6", had dark hair and only weighed 150 pounds.

As a full grown adult, I am 6'1", have sandy blonde hair and weigh 200 pounds. In his mind, because of the differences in our physical appearance, I had to belong to this other man. Of course, he didn't have any proof or any physical evidence to substantiate this claim, because it was all in his mind.

He then told me a story of how he was at Home Depot and some man—he couldn't even begin to identify—walked up to him and said, *"I know who you are. You're the man whose wife is having an affair with Tim."* My dad went on to say that he pushed this man up against the racks and picked up a cement trowel and was going to stab him in the throat with it, but the Home Depot employees tackled him and wrestled the trowel away from him, then escorted him out of the building.

Being in law enforcement for over ten years, I knew that if this had really occurred, Home Depot would have called the police, and he would have been arrested or, at the very least, cited for his actions. They wouldn't have just escorted him out of the building as if nothing had happened. I later contacted our local Home Depot and asked if there had been any altercations in their store in the past month, and they confirmed there had been no such incident.

After a couple of hours of listening to his arguments, I decided I didn't know enough about blood types to argue with him, but I did know that my mother was not having an affair with anyone. I explained to him that if he was that dead set on believing I was not his, I would pay for DNA testing to prove that he was wrong. This upset him because he could not be proven wrong; he was always right. How dare I have the means to end an argument about what he knew to be true?

My father never brought this up with any of my three younger sisters, even though he told me he believed all four of us belonged to someone else. It was just one more way for him to try to justify the fact that I wasn't the son that he wanted me to be. If I couldn't be like him and I couldn't do what he wanted me to do, then I must not be his. The DNA testing never took place because of what happened next.

Because he believed so strongly in the fact that my mom had had an affair, he became outraged and violent towards her. He threatened her life several times, destroying many things in the house. My mom was afraid for her life, and she would come down to my house in tears, shaking from fear.

My mother had also discussed her concerns with her religious leaders, hoping that they could do something or say something to my father to calm him down. I contacted them, and we talked about the discussion my father and I had earlier that week concerning his thoughts on my mom's infidelity. They were very taken aback and flabbergasted by the statement. They couldn't understand where my father could come up with such ideas.

One of the church leaders told me he would go over and visit with my father and see what he could do to try to calm him down and see where all of this was coming from. After he spoke to my father, he called me. I could tell by the tone of his voice he was upset. He said that when he went to the house, my father met him in the driveway with a 2x4 in his hand, holding it like a bat, slapping his other hand with it in a threatening manner. He said his eyes were vacant, and there was so much anger that he was afraid for his life.

I called several of my siblings and discussed the situation with them. I told them what my father had told me, what was going on with mom, and how he was acting toward her. I believed that we needed to seek medical intervention at this point. My siblings all agreed with me and asked what we needed to do next. I knew that we could have him committed to a mental institution based on his violent actions.

I contacted one of my friends who still worked for the police department in the city where my father lived, advised him of the situation, and asked to come by and take him to the hospital under suspicion of harming himself. My friend took my father in his patrol car, and my brother-in-law and I followed in our vehicle. One of the mental health care workers interviewed him, then came out to discuss the results with us.

She talked about all of his delusions and the individuals that he spoke of. She asked me if any of these people existed and I told her, to the best of my knowledge, these were all individuals that were in his mind. They committed him to the Behavioral Health Unit and said he would likely be there for six to twelve weeks.

He was formally diagnosed with paranoid schizophrenia and dementia. He was seen off and on in the unit for three months, where he received the proper treatments and medications to stabilize him. He was required to attend therapy twice a week to monitor his progress. Some sessions were only for him, others my mother would attend with him.

Things started to change between my dad and me after this. We still had our times of tension and disagreements; he still has a hard time admitting anything is his fault and the blame has now shifted from me onto my kids and my sister's children. But through everything, we have a better relationship than we ever have. It's hard at times for me to dismiss the past and understand his actions weren't always his. But I am working to let go of the anger and guilt.

20

Mothers And Sons

"When you are a mother, you are never really alone in your thoughts. A mother always has to think twice, once for herself and once for her child."

— *Sophia Loren*

My mom and I have always had a special relationship. I realize it's quite typical for mothers and sons to have a bond, sometimes even closer than their fathers, but mine was different because of my father. You've probably noticed that I sometimes refer to him as my 'Father' and other times as my 'Dad.' This is my way of separating his actions into two people:

Dr. Jekyll = Dad and Mr. Hyde = Father

My father was the sadistic bastard who punished me and created all of the horrible nightmares. My dad was the guy that I spent time with hunting and fishing, and gave me my sense of humor. My mom has always been my mom. I never referred to her as mother unless I was speaking formally. It's always just been *'mom.'*

For as far back as I can remember, my mom was always there, part of my life. She was the one who took us to school and picked us up. She was the one who dealt with the principals and teachers whenever I got into trouble. She went to all of my events, whether it was baseball, soccer, martial arts or scouting. She's the one that I always remember being there.

Since I learned to separate my dad and father, I've come to realize that my dad did help out with many of the scouting events as well. In fact, at one point my dad was the Scoutmaster. He was responsible for all of the scouting age boys in the entire neighborhood. I remember how everybody thought that it would be so great to have a dad who was over the scouting program. They thought that, as his son, I would have special perks and privileges that other scouts didn't. This was not true.

Throughout my life, during the times we were around other people, my *dad* was always present. When we were at home, it was my *father* whom I dealt with. Scoutmaster was just one more way for him to compare me or belittle me. My mom, however, was always so proud of me and always had a smile on her face whenever I accomplished anything. I was her only boy, and she made sure to tell everybody how proud she was.

My mom has always been more innocent and genuine than other people. She's not up on any of the current technology such as cell phones or Blu-ray players. She has a terrible time with it, just like we see depicted in the satire of the elderly. She's always been that way; not worldly at all. My mom approached everything in life with naive determination. Looking back now, I wish that life was still as simple as it was then.

Growing up in a household where the family's income was low, my mom always found ways to make sure we had what we needed. I talked earlier about wearing hand-me-downs from my sisters, and some of that is true. At times I would get clothing from my older male cousins, however, the remainder of my clothing my mom made. I remember she would even find patterns for Levi's and would buy denim at the fabric store and make homemade jeans for me to wear.

I was so proud of those jeans and they did look like everyone else's—at least from a distance. However, they still were not the name brands that were popular at the time, so they didn't have the special tags or other insignias on them that all the others kids pants had. So I was still made fun of because of my clothing. Incredibly, in junior high school I was even teased by one of the teachers in the school because of the clothing I wore.

My mom made shirts and pants for my dad and me and dresses for my sisters and her. There are countless pictures of my family together where we're all dressed similarly. My mom would spend months before Easter or Christmas, making clothes for all of us. My mom and sisters would all have matching dresses, and my dad and I would have matching pants and shirts. If you think of the way they dress on the television series, *'That 70's Show'*, that's very similar to the clothing we were wearing at that time.

Of course, it was never my mom's intention to make clothing that would bring mockery and ridicule to her children. She did a fantastic job, and it was impressive that she could spend that much time and could make something that we wore for years, not to mention the money that was saved.

One of my friend's mothers was fascinated by my mom's talent, and went to her for patterns and sewing advice. Many people couldn't believe her skill level. Some of my clothes that she made looked like something you would buy in the store.

There were a lot of kids in my neighborhood who had parents that could buy the designer brand clothes and nicer toys and bikes. If you were different, or didn't have the same things that everybody else had, you got teased. Kids are not always the most compassionate toward their peers.

A lot of the meals that we ate were created in a similar fashion to how she created our clothing; she would find things that she had in her pantry and somehow put them all together to make a meal. It wasn't necessarily a meal that you would expect—a lot of times it was a conglomeration of different items—but they turned out to be pretty good when they were all put together.

As an adult I absolutely despise macaroni and cheese. I want nothing to do with it, and I think it's probably one of the most horrendous meals on the planet. But when I was younger, my mother made a homemade version of macaroni and cheese that was fantastic. She melted three or four different cheeses together, made the macaroni and put it together herself. It wasn't from a box with fake, powdered cheese. My sisters and I have discussed how we miss that macaroni and cheese and how that was one of our favorite meals.

I also remember having certain brands of cereal for breakfast that none of the other kids I hung around with had even heard of. I later learned this was because certain foods were given to my parents because of their low income, similar to the WIC program today. Those foods could only be purchased or picked up through that program, which explained why none of the other neighborhood kids had them.

My mom always made sure we were fed and clothed. Come Christmas time we always had Christmas presents, and not just homemade gifts either. We received things that were just as nice as everybody else in the neighborhood. My mom would purchase Christmas gifts all year long for us. When she would have an extra $10 here or $5 there, she would spend it on presents for us. At the end of the year, we would have a lovely Christmas.

This was typical of my mom; she was always thinking of us first. She took care of the children and then she would worry about herself. I know it sounds cliché, but many times she went without certain things just to make sure that her children were taken care of.

Throughout my parent's marriage, my 'Father' showed up, and his anger and destructive personality were difficult for my mom because of her passive nature. It always seemed to be me that she would turn to for help and support. The older I became, the more she relied on me, as much as I relied on her. I was sometimes her only respite from the actions of my father.

My mom is very submissive and non-confrontational. To this day, she doesn't do well with conflict. Even between siblings, she would rather just hide and ignore what's going on instead of confronting it or dealing with it. At times this created a bit of an issue, at least for me.

There were several instances throughout my school years when I was having troubles at school. Sometimes it was with teachers and sometimes with bullies. Although I dealt with the bullies my own way. After being made aware of these struggles, she would grow angry. But being as passive as she was, she never confronted the problem or any of the teachers. It just wasn't in her nature.

When I was in high school, I had a teacher who did not like me. Probably because I was the class clown and pretty obnoxious, but no matter the reason, I was failing her class. Everybody who knew me just assumed that it was my fault; that I just hadn't turned in the work or didn't care to be there. However, in this case, none of this was true. I did do the work and I turned it in. However, sometime between me turning them in and having them returned to me, they would disappear.

My friend, Denise, was also in this class with me. She asked one day why I wasn't doing any work. She had noticed that I wasn't getting any papers returned from the teacher. By this time, I stopped finishing my papers because I wasn't getting them back even when I did turn them in.

I was failing the class, so my attitude was, *"If I'm going to fail even when I'm actually doing the work, I might as well not do the assignments at all."* After talking to Denise about the issue, she watched me do the assignment and turn the papers in. Once again, I didn't get them returned, and I was told I didn't turn them in. Denise decided she was going to help me with this problem.

She came up with a plan and when we received our next assignment, I made sure to complete it during class. When we both finished our work, I slipped my paper to her, and she placed it underneath hers and turned them both in. The following day our papers were returned and, as usual, mine was not. When I asked the teacher where my assignment was, she stated in a very condescending voice, *"You can't expect to receive a paper when you never turn in your assignments."*

Denise spoke right up, *"Excuse me. I know Shawn finished his assignment because I handed it in with mine."* You could have heard a pin drop. I think I might have even heard the sweat bead up on her forehead. The teacher grew scared, and she came up with an excuse as to why she could not find my paper.

I told my mom what was going on and that I was going to fail this class. I explained that I had done the work, and I even had friends helping me with turning in the assignments, but my teacher still insisted that I had not turned in any of the assignments.

Even though my mom always tried to be there for us, and I know she wanted what was best for us, she didn't know how to argue with the teacher over the assignments. The teacher just explained to my mom that I hadn't done my work, therefore I was failing the class, and my mom let it go at that.

I don't think that she believed her over me or that she looked at it as if it was my fault. She just didn't want to deal with the confrontation that she knew would occur with that teacher. She was afraid to push, and I don't blame her for that. It just wasn't her personality, and I can't condemn her for being who she is.

I eventually gave up, and quit going to that class altogether. I would spend the class time out on the football field playing Frisbee with the other kids that were skipping class. Or sometimes I would sit out in my car letting the sun warm me as I laid on the front seat. I would even sit in the hallway in the middle of the school itself. If I was stopped or confronted by one of the other teachers or administration, I would take whatever punishment that they decided I needed, rather than go to that class. At the time, I believed that if that's what they expected from me, that's what I was going to be.

Years later, after graduating with a Masters Degree, I talked to my mom about some of those previous school days and how I struggled. She apologized to me and told me that she wished that she would have pursued some of those a little further. She wished that she would have confronted more of the teachers and pushed me to do more of my work. She wished that she wasn't so afraid of everything, realizing how difficult it was for me.

She could see how well I was doing in college and how quickly I was advancing, and she realized that I could have started much earlier; that my high school years would have been much easier for me if she would have just been a little more aggressive with some of the people that stood in my way.

I tried to comfort her by letting her know that one of the reasons I had accomplished so much was because of those years of struggle. I had pursued education because of the hard times I had in school, and if she would have intervened, I may not have had that same motivation.

When I started performing stand-up comedy, my mom was one of the first people to be at the shows. She would sit in the front row and cheer me on. She has always been there, standing by my side, making sure I didn't back down, and that I followed my dreams.

After I had been performing comedy for about three months, I became a regular at the local comedy club. The owner of the club had allowed me to perform almost every weekend, but because I was still new, I only had 10 minutes of material. Every week, I was doing the same jokes. When I looked out into the audience, there was my mom, every single weekend, sitting on that front row and cheering me on while she listened to the same routine, week after week. She was always there, laughing even when I wasn't funny.

One particular weekend my family all came to the show; there were five or six of them that night at the club. This wasn't uncommon, because they would turn up on occasion with my mother to cheer me on, or to see the comic that was headlining that weekend.

As I got on stage and looked out into the audience, there they all were, sitting in a row, smiling at me. But this was different, because not only could I see *them*, but there was *my* face in the center of each of their chests.

My mom had taken my picture and had it screen printed onto t-shirts for all of my family members. They wore them to the comedy club to support me. It was the most awkward feeling in the world, to be staring out at my face looking back at me. I was trying to tell my jokes and keep my composure but it wasn't easy.

My whole family—right there for everyone to see—smiling and cheering me on just like a hockey game where I was the star player. I was extremely touched by their show of support and, at the same time, it was slightly embarrassing. I couldn't ask for a better family or a better mom. She was and is always there to show her love and support, no matter what.

To this day, she's been to every single show that she is capable of. She still laughs and applauds, and doesn't hesitate to let the audience know how proud she is of me and that I am her boy.

Now that my dad and I are closer and have worked through some of our problems from my childhood, he has also been to most of my performances. His medical issues sometimes keep him from attending certain events and shows, but he tries to be there just as much. We have reconciled and I love him dearly, but it's not the same close relationship that I have with my mom. I am honored and proud to call her – MOM.

21

Planes Trains And Automobiles

"When was the last time that you woke up and realized that today could be the best day of your life?"

— *Steve Maraboli*

I could never drive for a living. I guess I should be more specific. I could never be a long haul truck driver for a living. However, driving a dragster or a NASCAR would be a different story. *That* I could definitely do for a living. Being mostly blind and deaf means it would have to be a self-driving dragster, but give it a few years and this could be a possibility.

During my years as a comedian hypnotist, I had the great opportunity to visit most of the states. There are many years that I was on the road 48 weeks a year traveling from one state to another. Although I had some great times and I saw some beautiful sights, driving for 16-18 hours a day became very monotonous.

There were times that, after returning home from a long road trip, I wouldn't drive my vehicles to the store. I was so tired of driving that I just rode in the passenger seat. Now, I don't have a choice; the passenger seat is my permanent residence, which is really ironic. When you don't know what is in store for you in life, you have no idea what you might eventually miss.

Traveling was my opportunity to provide for my children and my family the things that were never provided for me. Sometimes I was able to take my family on these road trips. For 9 months of the year my children were in school and my wife worked full time, so we had to plan these trips around the end of the school year and vacation time for my wife.

We had some incredible experiences traveling to the different states, sightseeing and visiting monuments and museums in places that I had never dreamed of as a child. My children still talk about these trips. They were able to witness these things for the first time, just as I did, and it gave me an incredibly close bond with my children.

My children agree that their favorite memory from all of those years of traveling was their first trip across South Dakota. We were traveling on very limited funds. When we arrived at our first destination and checked into our hotel room, we were perplexed as to what we were going to eat that evening. We quite literally had about $25 to our name.

We drove to the local grocery store and purchased ramen noodles, bread, tuna fish and plastic utensils. We returned to the hotel room where we realized there was no microwave. But you know, sometimes you learn pretty cool things on the road. One of which is that if you don't put any coffee in the coffee pot, you get hot water. And Bam! That's how we made our Cup-a-Noodles.

It was one of the happiest times we had on the road. Here we were, broke in a hotel somewhere in the middle of South Dakota, having the best time of our lives. Eating coffee pot Cup-a-Noodles and tuna fish sandwiches.

My kids will talk for hours about their Dramamine induced hallucinations and the games that we made up to pass the time. Once we spent an entire trip making up new superheroes we'd like to see—giving them names and all their super powers. Other times, we played trivia games or word associations.

When I look back, it's not my graduations, accomplishments, my career or even my kid's accomplishments that I cherish the most.

It's those hours spent together traveling across this great country and surviving by any means we could. We are extremely close and love each other, but it goes beyond that. We also trust and help each other through all the hard times.

Every so often, we'd visit family in Iowa and Wisconsin. While there, we enjoyed a much easier and simpler life than the city where the kids grew up. The kids could run and play without worrying about any of the annoyances that urban life brings. We didn't live in a large city, but it was big enough that between the people and the traffic, it became frustrating. Stepping out of that for a little while and into the calm, peaceful atmosphere where my cousins lived, was a welcome change. While there, we would ride four-wheelers, shoot guns, have bonfires, and catch fireflies.

I know fireflies are commonplace for a lot of people, but to those of us who lived in a place without them, they were a rare and magical treat. They are nothing like the images that were portrayed in television and movies—okay, cartoons. The first time I ever saw them, I remember thinking I was having a seizure or mental episode, because suddenly, out of nowhere, came these streaks of greenish fluorescent light.

It was early enough in the evening that I could still see, but dark enough that I couldn't see the *actual firefly* that was leaving the glowing trail. As I looked out across the lawn, enjoying the evening, they started their dance of light and I believed I was malfunctioning.

My cousins who had seen this phenomenon occur every summer of their lives laughed hysterically as I tried to decide if I was in need of immediate medical attention. Here I was in my 30s and I felt like a small child in a wondrous land. My cousins marveled at my fascination with the little creatures as they lit up the fields and trees like a summertime Christmas light display. It was magical and I loved it.

My mom had traveled very little across this country. She had only traveled outside of Utah a handful of times—Texas to be with her sister, Arizona to visit her father and Wyoming for family reunions—and had not seen many of the different states or national parks and monuments that are beautiful and beloved.

For several years, after my busy season (usually spring and early summer), we would plan a trip with my parents so that my mom could visit some of the places she'd always wanted to see. By this time, my dad and I had reconciled a-lot of our differences. With his age and growth, along with my age and growth, things were no longer the way they used to be and he was an entirely different man than he was as I was growing up.

The first trip that I took my parents on was California. My dad had seen California when he was in the military, but he had never actually visited and spent time there. I took my parents through different sites and monuments; places they never would have been able to see otherwise. A couple of those places are especially memorable because of my mom. It was like watching a small child opening birthday presents every time we visited one of the locations she had waited her whole life to see.

We visited San Francisco and went out to the pier so she could see the ocean. It was her first time and she was overwhelmed by the vastness and beauty of it. She was also fascinated by the sea lions and other ocean life. We took her to do some shopping, to Ghirardelli Square to buy chocolates, drove down Lombard Street and saw all the sites that we could in in the time that we had.

We then visited Yosemite National Park. My mom has always been afraid of so many things, sometimes to the extent of missing out on life. I don't mean this in a cruel or harmful way; she has just always been extremely cautious about a lot of things. When it comes to the fight or flight response that every human being has, she has an extreme case of only *'flight.'* Basically, the exact opposite of me.

One of her greatest fears is heights. It has control over her and she refuses to go anywhere or do anything that might involve heights. When we took her to Yosemite, we visited one of the popular places known as Glacier Point.

Glacier Point is a viewpoint above Yosemite Valley. At an elevation of 7,214 feet, it's pretty high; especially for someone with a fear of heights. On the overlook itself, you can stare straight down a sheer cliff face, 3200 feet, to Curry Village, which is at the bottom of that cliff. The point offers a superb view of Yosemite Valley. Not only can you see Yosemite Falls, but also Half Dome, Vernal, Nevada Falls and Clouds Rest. If you have never been here I highly recommend it.

My mom was so nervous, we could see the fear in her face and her hands wringing. She was afraid for her life. But she didn't want the beauty and view to go to waste, knowing she would never again see these waterfalls, especially from this vantage point. She gripped my arm and together we walked right to the edge of the cliff. It was so impressive! She looked straight down to Curry Village and stood there while we took pictures in order to prove to the family that she really was right next to a cliff. In fact, after I took her picture, I took a picture over the edge, so they could see how far down it was, and how she had just conquered her fear. When you ask my mom what her favorite part of that trip was, she will tell you it was Glacier Point.

I believe that's probably the proudest I've ever been of my mom. I could name off a list a mile long of the things that I'm proud of about my mom, but that one tops them all. She overcame the biggest fear of her life so that she would not miss out.

My mom's fondest memory is going to Mount Rushmore. I have been lucky enough to go there several times with my family and even by myself while traveling through South Dakota. It's indescribable, and there's a huge difference between what you see in pictures or learn in school as opposed to what you see you when you're actually standing there, staring up at that mountain. It is one of the most awe-inspiring places I've ever been to in my life.

Because my mom had never seen Mount Rushmore, we wanted to make it an exceptional experience. During the day, we visited Crazy Horse monument and walked around the museum watching the different dances and shows that the Native Americans put on. We had a great day, and saw a lot of incredible sights. Mom was just like a little girl, fascinated by everything she saw.

My dad was in heaven! He'd always fancied himself a cowboy and at times in his life, he had been. He loved reading old westerns, he loved horses and when he was younger, he spent a lot of time in the rodeo.

For my dad, Crazy Horse was like living a dream. You could see him wander from display to display, looking at all of the memorabilia that was donated by the local tribes as well as the trappers and mountain man coalitions. I think my dad would have been perfectly happy just spending the entire time there, instead of visiting the other places that we had on our list.

We decided that we were going to visit Mount Rushmore in the evening so that we could watch the lighting ceremony. When it starts to get dark, there is an entire ceremony where the military retires the flag and they show a video of the history of Mount Rushmore. Then they turn on gigantic dazzling lights that illuminate the faces on the mountainside. It is extremely patriotic.

It was late August and the entire trip was warm and pleasant, until that evening, when a storm blew in and the clouds laid right on top of the monument so you could barely see the faces. The wind started to blow, and the rains began to come down. The temperature dropped about 30 degrees, but my mom was not going to miss a single moment. She sat in the rain and wind, waiting for that lighting ceremony.

I wasn't prepared for the drop in temperature or the rain. I was in shorts and a t-shirt, but I did my best to stand by my mom and shield her from the weather. As they prepared to start the service, it was as if Mother Nature stopped and waited for the ceremony. The wind that had been gusting up to 20 miles an hour stopped altogether. The rain ceased, the clouds cleared away from the mountain and the ceremony began.

I watched as tears filled my mom's eyes, and I, too, felt the pride and overwhelming joy that she felt. During the ceremony, they asked all of the veterans to come down on stage to be recognized. Although my dad was a Korean War veteran, he refused to go. I don't know if it's something that he would rather forget or if he just doesn't feel worthy of the recognition that comes with his service.

I may never know the reason for this. My dad will likely die with that secret. But his experiences, his sacrifices and his time in the military are some of the greatest gifts that any man can give to his country. I'm honored by him. And no matter what, I'm extremely proud of him.

22

Mistakes

"The person you care about the most is usually the person who you'll allow to hurt you the most."

— *Unknown*

Out of all the things that have happened in my life, this is the hardest for me to talk about, let alone write about. I have worried about how this book will affect my father and the relationship that we have now, along with the rest of my family and friends, because of the things I have written…things that I haven't discussed in my life until now. But the biggest worry and fear that I have is how it will affect my relationship with my wife.

On the outside, we always appeared to be the perfect couple and have been praised by our families and friends alike for the love and dedication we show toward each other. For 30 years, we have been together and struggled our way through what life had to offer. But there is a deep, dark secret that has haunted us for many years.

In this memoir, I have been honest with how I felt and the stories I have told. I know that there will be a fair amount of people who will be shocked and taken aback by my forthcoming attitude.

However, at this point in my life, I need to be honest, with myself and the world, about who I am, and accept the consequences.

There is something liberating about a terminal illness. My eyes have been opened to the fact that I can no longer live in denial or my make-believe world. My comic book hero days are numbered, and like all heroes, I must accept my actions and return to the realities of life that are sometimes not so pleasant.

"And above all, watch with glittering eyes the whole world around you because the greatest secrets are always hidden in the most unlikely places."

— *Roald Dahl*

When I fell in love with my wife, I couldn't see myself with any other woman. Ever. She was my moon and stars, everything I could ever love. However, sometimes human nature steps up to the plate, and things change. About nine years into our marriage, my attention wandered and I began a relationship with another woman.

I met her through a friend of mine that I worked with. It started innocently enough; talking about everyday things and life in general. However, it soon started down the path of creating an emotional tie that was getting stronger.

At first, our relationship seemed to fuel the fire for my wife, as it gave me a sense of someone else needing and wanting me. It was intoxicating. I was still fighting with my sense of self-worth and, even though I had a beautiful wife and two loving children, she made me feel desired on a new level. In my mind, she was someone who wanted me for me and not because she was obligated to me. I realize that these are my feelings, and I have taken responsibility for them.

After a few months, the relationship grew, and I found myself wanting to see and spend time with her more. My love for my wife had never faulted, but I was still infatuated with this new and forbidden experience.

As our attraction grew, I knew that if things continued on this way, it would lead to more than just an emotional relationship. I was totally lost, because I did not want to hurt my family, but my unconscious desire to be needed and wanted was too great to be ignored.

The inevitable happened, and we progressed further than just a friendship. It was not a full sexual relationship, but indiscretions happened. My wife was aware of my association with this woman, but did not know how far the relationship had progressed. After that moment of weakness, I was so full of guilt and self-hatred that I confessed my actions to my wife.

We always had a very open and communicative relationship. We had discussed everything in our lives from work to fantasies. We also decided that, as long as we could talk to each other and be honest, we could get through anything. We had even discussed the possibility of a situation like this occurring and determined that we could survive, as long as we were honest with each other.

When I opened up about my actions, she was devastated. I will never forget the look on her face. She was so destroyed that I believed our lives together were over. I had promised to love and honor her to the end of my days, but I had ripped open that promise and poured salt into the wound.

I pledged to myself that if we could get through this, I would never let it happen again. I never wanted to see her like that. It took several months, but we worked through some issues and became closer than we ever had. I felt as if I had walked through the fires of hell and survived to live and love again.

From that moment on, I promised that I would be honest and that my search for self-worth would be filled with my family. I would never again allow my shortcomings or weaknesses to steer my life. I began to feel like I needed to be tested to see what I was truly made of; to know what I wanted in life. However, I would soon find out how difficult this test would become. I had only seen the tip of the iceberg.

We had grown stronger and I had received forgiveness and compassion from my wife. I believed it was because I had been forthcoming and repentant. But I came to understand that it was actually because my wife was hiding secrets of her own.

At this point, I was unaware of a similar situation that was transpiring with her. She, also, had met someone, and that relationship was growing beyond what a friendship should consist of. Her increasing attraction to this man began around the same time as my transgression. Although I was open and gave a full disclosure of my relationship, she chose to continue to hide hers and did not take the opportunity to open up, allowing us both to move forward.

I initially suspected that it was more than a friendship after a couple of months, and I started questioning her about it. She adamantly stuck by her story that they were just friends and nothing else was going on between them. I had no reason to doubt her, so I accepted the answer and let it go. Time passed—a couple of years—and I became suspicious once again. Her interactions with him were growing, and she wanted to spend more time where he was and around him.

I started questioning her about her actions, but she deflected, saying I was just feeling guilty because of what I had done to her. At this time, I had been in law enforcement for several years, and I was not getting the answers I needed, so I turned to my skills as an investigator. It took several months, but I finally learned that they were much closer than just friends and their relationship was not simply platonic.

Once again, I confronted her about their relationship. I said that I knew what was going on, and told her that we could work through it. I said the only thing that would cause me to leave would be for her to lie to me about it. I gave her every opportunity to confess, but she still denied there was any type of relationship beyond friendship.

This sort of confrontation occurred for several years, but I eventually chose to believe that she had most likely stopped the relationship, and decided that it was best if it slipped into the past and we moved on with our lives.

About this time, I was chemically imbalanced because of my disease, but it had yet to be discovered. This imbalance, coupled with the knowledge that my wife was lying to me daily, put me on an emotional rollercoaster for the next several years. My depression was at an all-time high. I started to have nightmares and recollections of my earlier childhood abuse and, on top of this; I was overwhelmed with schoolwork, research and working full time. I will admit, I was not the most attentive partner, especially since my testosterone and hormones had decreased to the point of being almost nonexistent.

I stopped keeping track of whether or not she was still involved with him at this point, because I didn't care anymore. I was on the brink of taking my life just to get out of the misery that I was feeling. This was the lowest I had ever been. I didn't even feel worthy to breathe or take up space in this world.

I can't believe it, but this went on for six years while the disease grew inside of me like a tapeworm, consuming all of the nutrients from my body and leaving me starving; a hollow shell. Only this was an emotional tapeworm, and instead of destroying me physically, it was slowly eating me alive emotionally and mentally. My emotional state was so weak that I had no foundation to hold myself up.

After six years of living on the edge of a cliff and contemplating whether to jump or not, there was a reprieve; I was diagnosed with several chemical imbalances and started on some medication to regulate them. I became *me* again. It felt as if I had been reborn with a new purpose and desire. Cindee and I started our lives anew, and I felt alive once again. I was working hard at running the club as well as my career in comedy and schooling was becoming easier. The stress and emotional issues just seemed to melt away.

I believed that everything was great, and life couldn't get much better. But as we all know, sometimes when things get good that just means that the other shoe is about to drop—and drop it did. Looking back, I believe that ignorance is bliss—sometimes people shouldn't ask questions they don't want to hear the answers to. But that's not me.

For good or bad, I was a damn good investigator, and I knew something was not right. I started looking into the past few years and learned that not only did they not stop seeing each other, but they saw each other quite regularly. I now knew for sure that things between them were not going to change.

I once again confronted her—several times, in fact—both directly and indirectly about the two of them, and I always got the same answer; that I was paranoid and I needed to let it go. In all instances, she made me feel as if it was my fault entirely; that I was the one in the wrong and that she would never lie to me.

> *"With a secret like that, at some point the secret itself becomes irrelevant. The fact that you kept it does not."*
>
> *— Sara Gruen, Water for Elephants*

So I gave up and quit asking; stopped checking up on her and investigating the two of them. For several years, I had two thoughts; One: she was still coming home to me, and I still felt loved. Two: I would allow her to have what she needed because I apparently wasn't giving it to her.

I became a martyr. I felt broken and alone. But frankly I believed that I somehow deserved it. That my father had been right all these years, and I wasn't worth being loved. The one person who I believed would always be there and never hurt me was blatantly and, in my mind, maliciously lying to me.

My trust was broken. I stayed with her not because I made a promise to do so, or I somehow felt responsible, but because I thought that I couldn't do any better than her, nor did I deserve anything more.

As I started traveling to do comedy, I would be on the road for months at a time. I was away from home upwards of 48 weeks a year. I excused this by saying it was the only way to make money.

But, in reality, it was the only way I could escape the feeling of not being worthy of the truth. If I was home, I would have to look into her face and see the lies, day after day, and know that she was making a decision to hurt me.

This was also the reason I started to create all of the fantasy lives that I'd live while on the road. I told club owners, friends and fans tales of being an orphan and not having time for a family. I would elaborate by telling them the life of a traveling comic wasn't conducive to being in a relationship or falling in love. That part I believed. All of those made-up stories and lives were because I felt that my true self wasn't worth their time. I also knew that by being away, she had the opportunity to be with him. That was what she wanted, so I was giving it to her.

When the disease went into extra innings, and I lost my sight, there was a great deal of strain on us. I was entering a new world of darkness, and she was sitting by, helplessly watching it happen. It all became too difficult, and she turned to him for an escape. However, it was more than just an escape.

I had no more to give. I had lost my dignity, self-respect and my self-esteem. But more importantly, my faith and trust in the only person I ever wanted. And now to lose my sight? It was too much. I once again turned to an outsider for reassurance and company.

This was different than the first time, so many years before. I needed to know someone cared and loved me for me. She was there when I believed my wife wasn't. This relationship was based on caring and the desire to help myself as well as her.

The relationship became too consuming, and I realized I was not just abandoning my wife; I was losing my whole family. My children were at their wits end as well. They believed this woman was trying to take their father away. It took some time, but I found that I could not help her or me from where I stood. What I was losing outweighed what I could gain, so I ended our relationship.

I felt like my whole world had come to an end, and I confronted my wife one last time. I was very direct and even outright told her I knew about him and their affair. I received the same answer as always; the lie continued. That was it. The final straw. I couldn't take it any longer. I was tired of being lied to and treated like I was not worthy of her, so I left.

I told her that I had always tried to give her whatever she wanted, and for years given in and let her take what she needed. I conceded that I didn't deserve anything better. When I told her about my indiscretion, she asked me never to see the woman again, so I stopped that day. She became jealous of any friendship I had with any females, which would eventually cause fights between us. But still, she wouldn't give him up for me.

There is a story told about the great baseball player, Lou Gehrig. A reporter wrote of the incident: In New York, Lou came up to bat with two out in the ninth. The tying run was on third, and the winning run was on second. New York was one run behind, and a hit would either tie the score or win the game.

The count on Gehrig was three and two. The people in the stands were in an uproar. The pitcher wound up and delivered the third strike. It came smoking in, straight over the middle of the plate, and the umpire shouted, *"Strike three, you're out!"* Gehrig had not even moved his bat. Very slowly, Lou turned, spoke to the umpire, and walked to the bench. At that, the crowd went wild, for no one had ever seen Lou Gehrig argue with an umpire.

The reporters poured over the seats and out onto the field. They swarmed around the umpire and asked, *"What did Lou Gehrig say to you?"* The umpire smiled and yelled at Gehrig to come over. He said to Lou, *"Tell the boys what you said when I called the third strike on you."* Lou looked a little bewildered as he answered,

"Mister Ump, I only said, I would give ten dollars to have that one back."

The written story concluded with, *"There are people all over the world who would give ten dollars or ten thousand dollars to get just one minute back and for the privilege of changing something they said or did in that minute."*

MISTAKES

We all know that we cannot go back in time and change the past. I have said so many times, *"I just wish I could get a second chance at changing this situation,"* so I could right the wrong that I believed I had done. We cannot buy time, a past mistake, a lost opportunity, a hurting word...but we can experience forgiveness, and forgiveness starts within. We must forgive ourselves for our past so that we can have a future. With that forgiveness, we can begin again, we can be renewed, and we can live a happy, healthy life.

She has since stopped seeing him. We aren't what we used to be, but we're working on it. It has been a long road, and I wish I could say that I have forgiven her for the pain that this has caused.

I wish I could say that I have completely come to terms with the feelings that my father left me with—that I don't deserve to be treated better. The reality is that the best option I have is starting over. Dusting myself off and stepping back up to the plate, hoping for a chance to swing for the bleachers once again.

23
Go Straight To Grandkids

"And even if somebody else has it much worse, that doesn't really change the fact that you have what you have. Good and bad."

—Stephen Chbosky, The Perks of Being a Wallflower

My son and daughter are two very different people. I'm proud of both of them in their own ways. They have accomplished so much in their lives, and they have grown to be very responsible, caring adults with their families. Both of them are hardworking, honest, provide for their families and work at jobs that they love. I could not be more happy or proud of my children and the choices that they have made in their lives.

My son has always been the logical type. When he was five years old, he was regularly putting together 500 piece puzzles. When those were no longer a challenge he wanted 2,000 piece puzzles. He's always loved to read and would get lost in the imaginary superhero world, just like I did. He started to build Legos when he was very young, and still builds them, but in much bigger and more intricate designs.

My daughter is a very creative person. She has always loved to color and decorate. At three years old she wrote her first book, called *'Alligators are hard to catch.'* She drew different scenes on paper involving a zoo. After finishing the drawings, she told the story to my wife describing each scene. My wife then wrote her words on the pages for her.

When she was in 6th grade, she published a book titled, *'A world of stories'*. It's exactly as described—a book full of short stories that she wrote and illustrated.

This kind of creativity was typical for her throughout her entire life. It amazed me how well she could put on paper what was in her mind. She even drew the logo for our duck boat.

At 18 years old, my son decided that he needed to move out of the house and be on his own to make a life for himself. He moved into an apartment complex with two friends. His friends ended up losing their jobs and weren't able to make the rent. My son stuck it out; he worked hard and was able to pay rent himself. I told him that it would be okay if he wanted to move back in with us for a while, until he could get his finances in order. He said that he needed to do this on his own, and take care of himself.

He started dating and fell in love with one of the women who also lived in the same complex. She was 15 years older than my son, but he didn't care; he was in love. They dated for a couple of years and in August 2006, they were married. The two greatest things that came out of this marriage were her children from a previous marriage—a daughter and a son. Kylie was 14 and Justin was 12.

I have always given pet names to my family. My children and grandchildren were no exceptions. My son has always been *"Kid"* and my daughter *"Little One."* So it was only fitting that the grandbabies all got their own names. When Justin and Kylie came along, they were almost immediately given their names that have stuck to this day. Kylie is my *"Bug"* and Justin is *"Little Man."* Although he is not so little anymore.

I grew very close to those kids. Justin became my hunting partner when my son couldn't come with me. I took him shooting for the first time just weeks after I met him. He was a small boy, and the shotgun looked huge in his hands. At only 12 years old, he handled the weapon very proficiently, even though he had never held one before. As he grew, that ability grew with him, and he was a natural-born hunter and shooter.

The first time I took him, we went hunting ducks in the marsh. We talked about all of the safety precautions and proper hunting techniques. As we sat on the dike waiting for the sun to come up—it was still a half hour before legal shooting hours—we listened as the whistling wings of the ducks passed overhead. The last time I was this excited was the first time I took my own son hunting.

I remember that look on his face and how his smile just continued to grow bigger and bigger as the moments ticked by, bringing us closer to that magic hour when we could start shooting. I decided that when shooting hours started, I would let him shoot first and see how well he did before I joined in.

Just moments after we could begin, we saw a flock of ducks coming right at us. I pointed them out to him, and he started to get very excited. I calmed him down and reassured him that he would be okay, but to make sure that he picked out a single duck to shoot and not to go after the whole flock.

This is a common error for new bird hunters—they see the sky full of birds, point and shoot, thinking they surely cannot miss with the heavens so full. But the birds are flying 50-75 miles an hour, somewhere between 20 and 40 yards above your head, so it takes great skill to master. I remembered back to my first day hunting. I believe I shot 75 rounds into the sky and by sheer luck, might have hit one duck.

As the flock got close enough, I said, *"Go."* He raised the shotgun and fired...

Two shots rang out. Two ducks fell.

He had done exactly as I told him; he picked two ducks out of the flock, fired two shots and hit both birds.

For the next two hours, I didn't pick up my gun. Justin had filled his limit, and he had fired less than one box of shells. We started packing up, and I was so proud. It was his first hunt and he had proven himself. As we were leaving, I shot two more ducks, and we came home.

Every hunting trip that Justin and I went on was the same. He amazed me with his marksmanship and dedication to the outdoors, and he had the same respect for the animals as I did.

His sister, Kylie, also held a special place in my heart. When she was first brought into the family, we learned that she had scoliosis. She was going to Shriners Hospital where Tyler was taken so many years ago for his foot. I was always so proud of her because she did not let that slow her down or get in her way.

She studied dance and martial arts and she ran and jumped and played just like any other teenage girl. I was so impressed with her attitude and her ability to love life. We grew closer as we had what we affectionately called our Shriner lunch date. At this particular point in my life, I had a lot of free time. When Kylie would have her appointment at Shriners Hospital, I would take her there, sit with her through the doctor's visit, and then on the way home we would stop and eat lunch.

This was our time. We would talk about school and friends and anything else that happened to come up. It was very gratifying to me that she trusted me so much and could confide in me. On one particular lunch date, she was assigned by her school to take care of a baby for her child development class. It may not have been a live baby, but it acted just like one. The baby cried, needed to be fed, burped, and diapers changed just like a real baby.

On our lunch date, we had to take the baby with us. As we sat, we joked and teased about how everybody else in the restaurant was wondering about this 35 year old man and 16 year old girl with a baby. We speculated about all of the possibilities from grandfather to father and even to dating. We enjoyed every minute and even to this day, we laugh and joke about it.

We would go camping and on hunting trips as a family, and although Kylie never hunted, she would hike right along with us through the mountains or wherever we were hunting that particular season. She had the same love and respect for the outdoors; she wasn't about to miss it just because she was a girl. She got every bit as dirty, had just as much fun and went everywhere that we did.

When Tyler and their mother first got married, I believed that Tyler was rushing into it, but he was so in love that he didn't see it. I constantly told her that if she and Tyler ever got divorced, I got custody of the kids; once they're in my family, they don't get out. They just dismissed it as an empty promise. They had heard it all before. They didn't realize how much truth there was to my promise.

After two years of marriage, my son got divorced and Justin and Kylie moved to Ohio with their mother. I made it a point never to lose contact with them. I still tell people they are my grandkids. Because they are.

I am proud and honored to have them as part of my family. They have both grown into great adults. I am just as proud of them as I am my children. Kylie is now married to a wonderful man who takes good care of her. They have two sons, which means I have two great-grandsons, *"MJ"* and *"Tiny Might"*. I love telling people how I have six grandkids and two great grandbabies. Justin is in the Air Force, and I could not be more proud of the life that he leads.

My son remarried in 2013 to a beautiful young lady whom we just adore. She keeps him in line and works very hard. They have two darling little girls and I love them dearly.

My son and daughter-in-law's two girls I nicknamed, *"Happy Meal"* and *"Kamāmā."* They are such complete opposites, just like my own children. Happy Meal is always on the move and outgoing. She is boisterous and, at times, moody. Kamāmā was born with club feet just like my son. She has gone through casts and surgeries since she was a few days old and yet, she is so content and happy.

Arandalyn was married in October 2012. Our father-daughter relationship was typical of most. As a father, you'd like to handpick

GO STRAIGHT TO GRANDKIDS

the qualities you want in a son-in-law. Like all fathers and sons-in-law, there are a handful of things that I would like to kick him in the ass for, but overall, he takes care of my daughter and treats her like a princess.

They also have two children; a daughter and a son: *"Pooh Bear"* and *"Brick."* Pooh Bear is three and has speech problems due to loss of hearing that was discovered when she was two. She is making up for that now and talks up a storm. Brick is six months old at the time of this book, but just as happy and content as Kamāmā.

There are many things that, because of my disease, are tough and challenging on a daily basis. The inability to drive, watch hummingbirds or see a sunset. But absolutely nothing is as heartbreaking as not seeing my grandchildren's faces. The faces of the two oldest grandchildren are the only ones I was able to see fully sighted. Pooh Bear was a year and a half and Happy Meal was a year when I lost my sight.

I cannot describe the depth of pain I experience in not being able to see them as they grow, as they change and develop, knowing that the image that I see in my mind is what was left from before I lost my sight, and is no longer what they look like. I can make out ghostly shapes with dark spots for eyes and where their mouth is. I can tell if they're smiling or if they're looking at me, as long as I'm close enough to their faces. But from a distance, they are just another ghostly blur that blends into the background.

All I've ever seen of the two youngest is that ghostly image. I will never know what they look like; I will never see them grow and mature. Not only because of my vision loss but knowing that this disease is terminal, the possibility is very real that I will never see them graduate from high school, go on their first date, or get married.

This is, by far, my greatest fear and the thing that hurts the most. I have had a great life; I have seen many beautiful things. Witnessed the birth of my children and watched them grow into fine adults. I have traveled this great country; I have seen sights and locations that I never dreamed I would see.

I have had the privilege of being associated with some of the finest and most exceptional people on this planet. Even knowing what I will never have again, what I have lost and what I'm still going to lose; none of these losses compares to the knowledge that I might not be here for them as they grow.

I spend every moment possible with my grandchildren. Not taking a single second for granted, not putting off any longer what I have my entire life. They are everything I have, my will to live, my hopes and dreams. I know they will grow to be just as fine, upstanding and incredible as their parents.

Part 4
Why Not Me

24
TOO DUMB TO BE AFRAID

"This is the precept by which I have lived—Prepare for the worst; expect the best; and take what comes."

— *Hanna Arendt*

I have been told how brave I am; how well I have accepted this challenge, keeping my sense of humor about my condition. I think it comes back to a belief I've had my whole life—I'm just too dumb to be afraid. I can't say that, I wasn't afraid when this first happened. That I was going to lose everything I held dear and the activities that I loved doing. I was afraid that I was going to have to live the rest of my life in darkness, waiting for other people to help me.

However like most of the things in my life, when I'm told I can't do something, I take it head on and do exactly what I'm told not to. Because of all of the negative circumstances I've been surrounded with, I've learned if I want anything or to get anywhere in this life, the only thing to do is attack it. This behavior didn't change when all of my symptoms began.

I performed my act at an amusement park during their Halloween celebration for several years. They were some of the most memorable and fun shows I'd ever been a part of. They were rigorous and tiring, but the patrons of the park loved them. It wasn't uncommon to have over 1000 people at a single show, and I was doing three shows a day. The patrons could come and watch the show in between riding rides or visiting the haunted houses or any of the other festivities going on.

I loved this experience. But the best part was, since I was employed by the amusement park for that short time, I was allowed to ride all of the rides. I am a roller coaster freak—I love them! I've spent hours in line to ride new roller coasters in different parks. I've researched the tallest and fastest roller coasters in the world and been consumed with coming up with ways to get there to ride them.

Like flying, there are so many experiences on a roller coaster that are just indescribable. The speed, rapid descent, twists and turns—when all combined create a whirlwind of endorphins. Since losing my eyesight, I have returned to this particular amusement park to ride some of the roller coasters so that I could experience them in a new way.

It's amazing how different they feel and sound, now that I can't see. Having grown up near this park, I've ridden these rides hundreds of times throughout the years. To climb into them now, and hear the sounds and feel the rush of air on my face, gives me a whole new joy and thrill than ever before, especially not knowing what's coming next. It's like I'm riding it for the very first time.

Besides the fantastic roller coasters, one of the rides at this amusement park is a giant swing. Of course, when we hear the word swing, the mind immediately goes to a summer park or schoolyard where there is a 12 foot tall swing-set with a plastic butt-forming seat. You swing back and forth, kicking your legs as you lean, chain in hands, travelling a whopping ten feet per second.

However, *this* particular swing starts by strapping you into a harness made from heavy canvas and reinforced nylon straps that are much like a sturdy pair of overalls.

As it begins you're pulled by a cable to the top of the launch tower which is 150 feet above the ground. (I find it hilarious that as you stare down at the ground below you, there is a small kite-string-thin net that is meant to catch you if things go wrong.)

When you're ready, you pull the ripcord, releasing your harness from the original cable that hoisted you to the top. There is a moment of free falling—a fraction of a second, but long enough to be the most frightening yet exhilarating experience—before the swing cable catches and you start the arc toward the ground. It's at this moment that you are looking at that netting praying to God it will save you before you splatter on the cement below.

Reaching speeds up to 80 mph—roughly 118 feet per second—it's a feeling akin to skydiving, or swooping along the ground in a hang glider. Then, like a pendulum, you swing in the opposite direction 100 feet into the air and then back and forth until your momentum has died down enough that you can get back onto the platform.

The ride itself isn't the part that I am too dumb to be afraid of; I've ridden the ride several times. But after I was diagnosed with my heart condition, I was told not to participate in any strenuous or highly excitable activities that could put undue stress on my heart. As usual, me being who I am, I didn't listen.

At the entrance to the ride, there was a sign that was about eight feet long and five feet tall with great big bold letters that read, *'DO NOT RIDE THIS RIDE IF:'* and directly below that, *'YOU HAVE ANY HEART CONDITION.'* It went on to list other cautions, but I focused on those words alone.

I read it over and over, *'ANY HEART CONDITION.'*

A typical person would probably agree that this ride would most definitely add excess stress. I read it and thought to myself, *"I wonder why?"* and bought myself a ticket to ride.

My wife was with me at the time, and she was extremely nervous and frightened for me, knowing that I had just gone through several episodes of what can only be explained as similar to a heart attack.

But she said she knew there was no stopping me, so she might as well just let me go. If I died, at least I was doing something I loved.

As they connected me to the cable that drew me to the top of the swing, I could feel the exhilaration spike and my heart start pounding. With an oversized heart, it felt like it was going to pound right out of my chest. Like there was a man inside of me beating on my ribcage with a hammer trying to escape. One of my best friends was next to me and said he could also feel my heart as it pounded through the harness that held onto the both of us.

As we reached the top of the tower, I could feel the adverse effects of the stress. I was light headed and starting to get tunnel vision, as my heart worked overtime to pump blood through my body. But as always, I looked fear straight in the face and pulled the ripcord.

As we dropped from the sky into the freefall, my heart stopped. For the first time, I thought to myself, *"Dear God, what have I done?"* Then, as we started to swing towards the ground at that high rate of speed, I realized that I was going to live! My heart was still beating, and I was very aware of the rush that I was feeling.

I screamed at the top of my lungs and laughed uncontrollably, not with fear or pain but pure adrenaline. I felt completely overjoyed with the thrill of that ride. I had faced the dragon and with the slash of my mighty sword, slew him and reaped the rich rewards.

I have not had the opportunity to ride again since I lost my eyesight. However, I'm looking forward to returning to the park so that I can appreciate that as well.

I want to continue to experience things, even though they may be dangerous and, I'll admit, probably not the smartest ideas. The craziest of these is driving. There's nothing more aggravating than not being able to drive yourself to the places you need to go and have gone with such ease before. I've learned to get around with my cane, the bus system and other means, but 90% of my transportation from home to doctors, physical therapy or even my shows, is dependent on somebody else.

I hate asking for help in any way, and asking for rides tops my list. The people who drive me around the most are my family and close friends. They really don't have a problem with it, and they wouldn't have offered if they didn't want to do it, but it still makes me feel like I'm putting them out, or keeping them from other obligations they may have. However, there are no other alternatives at times.

When I decided to go hunting again after losing my eyesight, I knew that it would be difficult for me to get into some of the locations where we hunt. Some areas are rugged, treacherous and steep.

As an example, on one of the mountain ridges where we hike, you can stand on top and see both sides simply by looking over one shoulder then the other. The apex of that mountain is quite honestly only two or three feet wide, with almost vertical drops down both sides.

We affectionately call this place, *'The back side of hell.'* It is so treacherous and yet so beautiful; it draws you in like sin. And just like that transgression, once you get to this location, it is extremely difficult to get back out. Nonetheless, it's where most of the deer are found. So fear doesn't keep us from venturing there.

Several months before one deer hunt, I purchased a side-by-side so that I would have better access to some of those locations. A side-by-side is a recreational vehicle similar to a four wheel drive buggy that drives like a car. It has two or four seats, depending on the model.

The purchase itself is ridiculous if you think about it—I bought an off-road vehicle to get places in the mountains that I could not hike to because I am blind—which also means I cannot drive the vehicle I just bought.

When we unloaded the side-by-side from the trailer for the first time, it wasn't me who got to drive it. I must say, it's a unique feeling to purchase something, knowing that someone else is always going to be using it to drive you around. It almost makes me feel like a very wealthy person who has purchased a high-class limousine and hired a chauffeur. My side-by-side was my limousine, and my chauffeur was my son-in-law. But being in my own seat with a seatbelt and having bars to hold onto in case the ride got rough was a much safer option.

We drove around for two days scouting deer, having fun and seeing what the vehicle could do, since it was new to both of us. As we sat in camp one day, soaking up the mountain air and sun, I thought to myself, *"That's my side-by-side, and I'm going to drive it."*

You know those ideas that, right after you have them, you think to yourself *"This is foolish, but it's going to be fun."* And we have all heard the running joke about rednecks saying, *"Hold my beer and watch this!"* Yeah—this was one of those ideas. The fact that I could only see about five feet in front of me and that vision was obscured and I had no center vision to speak of didn't matter to me at the time. It just sounded like a great idea.

Let's put the blind guy behind the wheel of a high-speed off-road buggy and watch as he attempts to drive it through the mountains. Hopefully without running into any trees, rocks or large animals. And to help guide my way, I will simply hold my cane out the window.

Of course, this was a joke; not the driving part, but having my cane out the window. I should specify. I don't mean that I didn't hold my cane out the window as I drove, but the joke was I thought it would be hilarious to video a blind guy driving a vehicle with his cane out the window, using it to guide his way as I do when I walk around.

Just to ease your mind a little bit, I'm not *completely* stupid. The keywords to this phrase are *'Not Completely'*. Almost, but not entirely. I had my son-in-law line up the side-by-side so that it could go in a straight line down the center of the roadway without running into anything. Well, at least for a short period.

That period was approximately 100 yards. At the end of that 100 yards, he informed me, there was a large stand of trees that would stop me before I could drive off the cliff. I made sure that all of the animals and other pedestrians were out of the way as my son-in-law stood to the side of the road with camera in hand as I made my first attempt of driving under the influence of blind.

When I bought it, I discussed with the salesperson how crazy it was for a blind guy to be purchasing this vehicle. He wanted a picture of me driving it so that he could post it as a joke to show other people at the shop. As we laughed at the stupidity of it, we all believed that it was just that—a joke. At most, he thought I would just sit in the driver's seat posing for a picture that he could use as a conversation starter with other customers.

I climbed into the side-by-side, strapped myself in and started the engine. I waited for my son-in-law to give me the all clear; I stuck my cane out of the window and stomped down on the accelerator. As the vehicle lurched forward, I immediately started tapping my cane back and forth like we are trained to do when walking.

Obviously, it was doing me absolutely no good. The front of the vehicle was still three or four feet in front of me, but it made for a hilarious sight. The buggy bolted forward down the road, and I passed my son-in-law at the blazing speed of about 10 miles per hour. In my mind, I may as well have been in a military jet, as I felt the acceleration once again. As I drove past him, I was screaming at the top of my lungs with excitement, adding some drama to the video.

When I had traveled what I believed to be 75 yards or so, (I really had no idea exactly how far it was; it just felt right) I put my foot on the brake to stop rather than slamming into the stand of trees. It was the most incredible feeling. Driving had always been more of a necessity for me. Almost bothersome. Until I could no longer do it.

Those few yards of driving—the pure exhilaration of feeling the vehicle moving and me being in control of it—whether I could see what I was doing or not doesn't change the fact this was one of the fondest of my new memories.

I haven't attempted to drive any other vehicles since. However, I am planning on driving more, whether in a big open field, on a straight away, or even just back and forth in a parking lot where I know that I cannot hurt anything.

Both of my kids have volunteered to go with me. Whether they're sincere or teasing, I never expected anybody to want to ride with me, but it's frightening how many volunteers I've had. It just goes to show that I'm not the only roller coaster freak in my family.

25

Dogs Are The Best Medicine

*"I'm suspicious of people who don't like dogs,
but I trust a dog when it doesn't like a person."*

—*Bill Murray*

Dogs have always been a vital part of my life. When I was younger, there was always a dog around the house. From Dachshunds to Spitz and all types of mutts in between, we always had a dog. The first dog I remember was a Dachshund we named Tinker.

Tinker was the typical Dachshund; the rusty brown color, long and thin with short little legs and a long pointy nose. She was the perfect family dog. She loved to run and play and cuddle. I don't remember a lot about Tinker because I was very young, but I do remember one day we woke up, and Tinker was gone. My father told us they thought she just ran away; we tried finding her, but we never saw her again. Later, we learned that they took her to the vet and had her put down because she was old and had many medical problems.

The dog that I remember most was a breed called Spitz. We got her as a pup, and we named her Candy. She was about the size of a lab, pure white and had very long fluffy hair. Candy and I were best friends, and whenever I would get into trouble or needed alone time, I would go out and climb into her house with her.

Candy was my first therapy dog, even though I didn't realize it. She was always there for me when I needed an escape, when I just needed to talk or play. She was always there to lick my face, cuddle, play fetch or just sleep side by side. Even in the middle of winter, I would go out and climb into the doghouse with her whenever I needed that escape.

Candy spent all of her time in the backyard. We had a large yard, and she had a big dog house that was warm in the winter and cool in the summer. Candy was my responsibility; I fed her and cleaned up after her. I would go out periodically and clean out her house and add new straw for her to stay comfortable.

Candy had her first litter of puppies when she was only about a year old. Instinctively, she dug a hole underneath some of the shrubbery in my parent's backyard to have the puppies. Even though she had the dog house, her instincts took over and she prepared her own place. She had them sometime during the night and we didn't even know that the pups had been born until we could hear them whining underneath the bushes.

When I found the puppies, I climbed underneath the bushes and retrieved them. We made sure they were all washed up and healthy and placed them in the dog house where they could be comfortable. It was clean, safe and Candy could go in and out to take care of them. I was excited because of the new puppies to play with, but a little disappointed because I had lost my place of escape.

For the next couple of days, I would go out and check on the dogs to make sure everything was okay. One day, I noticed that she was having some issues, she would shiver and almost convulse periodically. She had stopped taking care of the puppies, and we could tell that she was in a lot of pain. I realized while I was checking her that there was something wrong with her fur. I could see things crawling around.

I looked closer and realized there were maggots in her coat. None of us had realized that the flies were bad and that they had laid eggs on her after she had delivered the puppies. The eggs hatched, and they were eating into her body, so she was in excruciating pain.

We contacted a vet, and they told us the best thing for us to do was to shave her fur as close to her skin as possible, dilute some iodine in water and coat the affected area with it. My mother and I used scissors and an old set of hair clippers and shaved her coat down as close as we could to the skin. We could see where all of the maggots had burrowed into her. We poured the mixture onto her body, and she whimpered in pain, but she never moved. Immediately all of the maggots came out of her body, and we were able to pick them off.

We had to take care of the puppies as well. I took it upon myself to care for them during her recovery. I bottle fed them for weeks and I would stroke them and clean them. I would make sure they stayed warm during the night and cool during the day. I took care of Candy, making sure that I kept the wounds clean and there wasn't any infection. After a week, all of her wounds had scabbed over, and she was acting like a mommy dog once again, taking care of her puppies.

We had Candy for about 10 years. One evening, we came home from a night out and I could hear her crying in the yard. I found her lying in the middle of the lawn; she looked up with those puppy eyes, happy to see me but not able to move.

She tried to stand several times, but her back legs just wouldn't work. My father wanted to put her down, but I begged and pleaded with him to take her to the vet—I needed her, she was my dog. I believe, for the first time in my life, he did something I asked. When we got to the vet, they were just closing, but they allowed us to come in.

After a brief evaluation, it was determined that her back was broken. No one knew how this occurred; there were many assumptions and speculations. But the fact of the matter was, I was going to lose my dog.

This was the hardest thing I ever had to go through up to that point in my life. I finally had something that made me happy and gave me solace. She loved me as much as I loved her and I cried for weeks after we left the vet's office. I felt like I would never have another bond with anyone or anything like I did with her.

I wouldn't allow my dad to get rid of the doghouse and for years, I would climb in and spend hours by myself crying and wishing that I had her back. We had several other dogs after Candy. However, as much as I loved all of them, I never had the bond like I did with her. Fortunately, that eventually changed.

I had been in law enforcement for about two years when I approached the city about sponsoring a canine. One of my good friends was a canine handler for another agency, and I had been assisting him in training some of his dogs. He helped me find a dog to train for myself and that dog became one of the greatest friends I've ever had in my life.

I found my dog by accident. His name was Baron Von Aesch. I was looking for a canine to train because purchasing one that was already trained was around $6,000. I saw an ad for a two year old purebred German Shepherd for sale.

I decided I would look at the dog even though I knew I probably couldn't afford what she would want for him. I drove about an hour south of my home to visit with the owner. I instantly fell in love with the most beautiful German Shepherd I've ever seen in my life.

He had great drive and was obedience trained. He was brought over from Germany as a puppy, and he had a pedigree as long as my arm. Baron understood commands in English, German, and Spanish. His owner told me that she'd always wanted a pedigree dog, and she had paid $8,000 for him, including shipping from Germany. She was only asking $2,500. She had some medical issues and was moving into a condominium that didn't allow pets.

I told her I was looking for a dog that I could train for law enforcement purposes, but I was doing it on my own, and I would have to pay for everything out of pocket. I was heartbroken that there was no way I could come up with that much money, and I had to walk away from an amazing dog.

I left and was resolved to continue looking for another dog. The next day I received a phone call from Baron's owner. She told me she was so impressed with the way I handled Baron and how he bonded with me. She wanted to donate him to me for the training. I wasted no time in driving to her home a second time.

We trained between two and four hours a day, four days a week. He learned faster than any of the other dogs in the training. He eventually started teaching himself, picking up on things the very first time we did them.

Baron and I nationally certified as a narcotic detector team, and he was certified to detect ten different substances. Twice in my career, I was offered $10,000 for him by other agencies because of his capabilities but there was no way I was going to sell him; he was like one of my children.

My friends were just as impressed by him as I was. They would come over to the house not to see me, but to play with Baron. Besides drugs, one of the things we trained for was searching for articles. These items could be anything from a ditched weapon to stolen or lost articles, or even finding people.

When I certified him in article searching, the instructor took us to a park where children and families played. We left Baron in the back of the vehicle, and we talked for a few minutes. He said that to certify, Baron would need to find a particular article in less than three minutes.

We had been training for years to do this, and I had a plethora of different items to choose from. This wasn't good enough for the instructor. He took his wedding ring off of his finger, showed it to me, and promptly threw it out into the middle of the park. I was completely shocked and horrified.

All he said to me was, *"Your dog has three minutes to find my ring, and if he doesn't, you owe me a new one before I go home to my wife."*

I was slightly worried at this point. I had all the faith in the world in my dog, but I'd never had anybody trust us that much. It took Baron one minute and thirty seconds to find that ring.

Because of this skill, when my friends would come over, they would throw loose change, necklaces, keys and sometimes their wedding rings into the yard just to see how long it would take Baron to find them. I'm proud to announce that we never lost a single article.

But Baron wasn't just an incredible narcotics detector dog and evidentiary dog, he was also the best babysitter we'd ever had.

When my children were young, and they would play out in the yard, he would sit on the porch and watch them. He would never leave the porch unless he believed they were in trouble; mostly he would just watch them play.

Once, we were on a trip with my in-laws and my wife's sister's family. We were camping along a river where we loved to fish and would make several trips there during the summer.

One afternoon, my brother-in-law and I were sitting outside the campers enjoying the sunshine and breeze, when Baron came up to me whining and nudging me to get out of the chair. Since I was camping and relaxing, I ignored him and told him to lay down. Baron ran off into the bushes, and a few moments later, came back again to whine and nudge me.

I continued to ignore him and was getting annoyed because I was relaxing and I didn't want to play. After this went on for several minutes, he finally grabbed one of my pant legs and started to drag me out of the chair. Like a sledgehammer to the forehead, I realized there was something he really wanted me to see. Yeah yeah—I know!

As I stood up, Baron ran down the trail toward the river, and I followed him. As I cleared the bushes and could see the river, I watched Baron grab my little two year old niece by her diaper and drag her back away from the river. She had wandered off and nobody had noticed, except Baron. He was trying to tell me that she was too close to the river, and he knew she shouldn't be.

When I blew him off, he would run down to the river and drag her back as far as he could, then come to alert me once again. I finally responded, finding that he had saved her life. I never ignored him again; he proved that he was much smarter than I was and that he always had a reason for what he was doing.

People who didn't get to experience Baron have a hard time believing some of the feats that he could accomplish. In fact, even people who witnessed his abilities had a hard time believing. On that same camping trip, we were sitting around a fire late one night, talking about Baron and how he knew he needed us to help with my niece.

We talked about some of the other things that he had accomplished in the past few years. My brother-in-law and father-in-law could not believe some of the things that I was bragging about regarding my dog. I told them how he could pick up a scent as small as a penny in a field of alfalfa. Of course, they didn't believe me, and they wanted proof.

I asked my brother-in-law to pick up a rock, just any ordinary rock. However, it needed to be distinguishable from any other rock. He found a rock that had a small chunk taken out of it that made it look like it had a smile. I told him I didn't even want to touch it or see it, I just wanted him to throw it as hard as he could up the side of the mountain that was in front of us.

It was late at night, and it was dark; he looked at me as if I had lost my mind, but he threw that rock as far up the mountain as he could. We all heard it hit amongst all of the other rocks on the mountain and then all sound stopped. He looked at me and jokingly asked, *"Now what, your dog's going to bring that rock back?"* I said, *"Not yet,"* and we continued laughing and talking as Baron sat patiently right beside my chair. Eventually they all forgot about the rock.

After about 30 minutes, I looked at Baron and gave him the command to search. Baron took off from camp like he was on fire and headed straight toward the mountain.

Everyone looked at me as if I was crazy, thinking there was no way he would be able to find that rock now, especially with so much time having passed. I just poked the fire with a stick and kept talking, carrying on the conversation that we were having.

They were unaware that Baron had returned and was sitting next to my chair once again. I lowered my hand down below his mouth and gave him the command to *"drop it"* and the rock fell into my hand. I didn't even look at it; I just gave it to my brother-in-law and asked, *"Is this your rock?"* Everyone around the campfire could not believe that he had just retrieved the exact rock.

I could write an entire book on his abilities and the amazing stories; how he found drugs, lost articles and even tracked criminals that had run from the scene of a crime. I spent more time with him than I did with my own family, and I became very attached. Between training and working, we were together 12-15 hours a day.

He was a very special animal, but as we all know, animals don't live as long as humans. Baron lived to the age of 12, which is pretty old for a working dog. He was becoming blind and deaf, and he ended up with some internal bleeding. The hardest decision I've ever had to make in my life was to relieve him of all of that pain and suffering. There isn't a day that goes by that I don't think about Baron, his faithfulness and the amazing things he could do.

As amazing as Baron was at searching, narcotics detection and as an all-around companion, my next dog was just as talented at hunting and retrieving, and he became the therapeutic dog that Candy had been for me.

Dozer is a purebred Black Lab. Even though I wasn't looking for a new dog, I found him. It had been two years since I lost Baron and I didn't think I could ever have another dog. We were at a family reunion in a small town in Idaho, and we stopped at a gas station for some drinks.

I saw a poster advertising Black Labs for sale and called the number. I got the address, and we decided to stop and just look at the dogs. I had no intention of getting a dog; it was still tough for me to even think of another dog after Baron.

When we arrived at the home, there were 11 puppies. Two of them had already been spoken for, so we looked at the other nine. We were utterly beguiled by two of them—both males and as different as they were the same. When we got them home, we named one Dice and the other Dozer. Dice had slick black hair and a narrow face, where Dozer had a long flat coat, a more blocky face and weighed 5 lbs more than his brother.

Dozer got his name when we fed him the first time, and he pushed his bowl across the floor like a bulldozer. I spent the next year training them in hunting and obedience. Dice never turned out to be a hunting dog because he was gun shy, but Dozer was incredible.

As quickly as Baron taught himself how to search and find drugs, Dozer was the same with game smells and finding downed birds. It didn't matter what kind of bird either; we hunted pheasants, grouse, chukar, ducks, and geese; they were all the same to him. He had a nose that was unbelievable.

When he was only a year old, we took him goose hunting for the first time. My son shot his first goose on this hunt, and I was so proud to be there. We were hunting late in the season; the pond was frozen, and there was snow on the ground. The goose flew about 200 yards out over the ice and then fell. Dozer was still young and didn't see the goose fall, so he didn't realize that he needed to retrieve the fallen bird.

I walked him over to the edge of the ice where he could see the black feathers contrasted on the ice, but he was unsure of what I wanted. I walked another 50 yards out and pointed out the spot once again,

Dozer immediately perked up and started pulling against me; I let him go, and he bolted across the ice toward the goose. As he approached the goose, he realized it was almost as big as he was and he had never retrieved anything so large.

He slammed on the breaks and dug his nails into the ice, sliding to a stop about 20 feet from the goose. He looked back at me as if to say, *"Are you shitting me!"* He circled the goose twice before building up enough courage to sniff it. I was continually giving encouragement like a personal trainer at a gym. *"Come on, you can do it! Get it! Get it! Get it! Good Boy!"*

The smell was familiar, so he attempted to pick it up, but it fell out of his mouth because it was so large. He eventually got a hold of it and brought it back, proud as a peacock strutting the whole way. He since has retrieved many geese and even several swans without even a hesitation.

A year later, my daughter rescued a third Black Lab. We were celebrating my parent's 50th wedding anniversary at my sister's house. Her neighbors had several puppies that were out on the back deck of their home. They were barely six weeks old, emaciated and a few had fallen off the deck; one even died because of the fall.

My daughter went to their door and asked if she could take the puppies, and they were glad to be rid of them. We brought them home, nursed them back to health and found proper homes for them, all except one.

She had fallen in love with the only female puppy, and there was no way we were giving her away. She named her Odee. She has an incredible drive when she wants to show it. More than not, though, she just wants to give you her love and be loved. She will never be a hunter. She's our cuddle-bug, and she seems to know exactly when we need her attentiveness.

I reached a point in my life where, once again due to this disease, I was experiencing some major depression. I was struggling with suicidal thoughts and daily depression. My disorder threw my hormones completely out of whack. My testosterone level, thyroid hormone, and others were extremely low, along with the situation with my wife and our marriage. I was struggling every day, spending hours sitting alone, surfing the internet and otherwise being a recluse.

One of the things that kept me from committing suicide was my love of hunting with my dog. Many times I allowed the most drastic of thoughts to go through my mind, and the only thing that stopped me was the thought of being with Dozer. There were days that I would just take Dozer and go to the nearest marsh or mountain where we'd spend all day hiking or just sitting. We'd sometimes get game and other days I would not even fire a shot.

On those days we may have seen the game we were after, but I had no desire to shoot. I just wanted the time away from everything, watching Dozer work. It would refill my emotional well, walking around in the crisp mountain air, with that smell of the woods and the crunch of the ground beneath my feet. I would stop and just listen as he would run through the woods, back and forth, following the abundant smells that were surrounding him.

Sometimes we'd walk around the dikes that held the marshes separate from the Great Salt Lake. Most people don't appreciate the marsh—the salty air and the stagnant waters make for an interesting odor, but it's like cologne for me. The combination of waters and grasses, cattails and other growth are a beautiful contrast against the fall and winter sky. The view, combined with seeing my Dozer full of energy and excitement, was enough to make me want to continue living.

I know that some of you may be thinking, 'That's ridiculous.' But I've learned throughout my career and education that when it comes to suicide and depression, it doesn't matter what keeps you here, as long as it keeps you going and you use it to continue your life. For me, that thing was hunting with Dozer.

For the longest time, it bothered me. I wondered why hunting was the thing that kept me here; not my family, my wife or my children, but hunting? The thought that, if I ended my life, I would never be able to hunt again.

I was troubled tremendously by this. It wasn't that I didn't care about my family or even that I thought they would be better off. Plain and simple, when I was in this state, I didn't think about them at all. I didn't reflect on how they would react. I didn't think about how they would feel. I didn't think about the fact that they would be better or worse off without me.

If you have never been through this type of depression; being on the verge of ending it all, it's hard to understand. You don't think of anything—it's just a hollow, empty space where all I thought about was how miserable I was, and I wanted a way out. Every time those feelings came to me, the only thought that took them away was going hunting with Dozer. I realize that is what all of the dogs in my life have been—I wasn't there to take care of them, they were there to take care of me.

26
Lost But Not Forgotten

"Don't focus on what's gone, focus on what's here."
— *Shawn Paulsen*

It is believed that our dreams are the unconscious mind's way of getting rid of the cluttered and stressful thoughts that we have, giving us temporary relief from that stress. Typically, blind people see transportation as a very stressful thing, and it creates panic in some. Interestingly, I read a study where a high percentage of people who went blind after having sight dreamt about trains. I, however, dream of flying.

Not Superman flying, although that would fit my *'living in a comic book'* mindset, but actual flying. For as long as I can remember, I have wanted to fly. There is nothing like the experience of sitting behind the controls of an aircraft and leaving the earth and all your worries behind. The sky is beautiful and so clean when you're above all the commotion and smog of the city. It's where you can be at peace and just enjoy life for what it is.

I can still remember the first time I ever flew. It was when my wife and I took our first trip out of the country. We were invited by friends to go to Mazatlan, Mexico. Up until then, I had only left the state of Utah a handful of times, and that was mostly just family reunions to Wyoming.

We were 20 years old and had two small children, but we decided to use our income tax return to go. Our friends and family all told us that we needed to save our money, or use it to purchase a home, or for the children. But we decided this was an opportunity that we may never experience again and, in retrospect, I am glad we did.

We arrived at the airport on a cold day in February. We were delayed for several hours because our airplane was damaged by a luggage cart. After a long wait at the airport terminal, we finally boarded the flight and were off.

The flight was exhilarating and even though I had an aisle seat and could not see outside of the aircraft, I was happy as a pig in shit. I knew as soon as the airplane started down that runway that I was going to have to do this more.

We arrived in Mexico and loaded onto an old bus that was reminiscent of the hospital buses used on the television series M.A.S.H. It made school buses seem like riding in a luxury sedan.

If you have never been to one of the tourist areas of Mexico, I'll try to explain it to you. As we traveled through the city towards our hotel, I was shocked and disappointed with what I saw. The poverty and meager way of living were appalling and heart-wrenching. I couldn't believe that we had wanted to come here so badly, and this is what we found.

I wanted to leave and go back home where I was comfortable and felt safe. Then in just a blink of an eye, we crossed over into what the residents affectionately call the *'golden zone'*. It was like we were with Dorothy and had just traveled to Oz. We had been in a black and white barren wasteland and now everything was colorful and bright. I just kept waiting for the wicked witch to show up and chastise us for dropping in unannounced, but that ruby slipper never dropped.

I remembered a movie I had watched years ago; Running Scared. A couple of the actors went on a vacation and saw hundreds of people standing still, looking out into the distance. They asked what everyone was looking at and were told, *"The Sunset"*. They didn't believe that people would take the time out of their day just to watch a sunset, but by the end of their vacation, they were joining in, watching this beautiful scene and realizing that there are no two alike.

We walked from our hotel to the beach that very night and watched the sun set into the ocean. This was the first time my wife or I had ever seen the ocean, and it was beautiful. I can still see myself sitting on the beach, watching that bright red sun as it descended into the water. Witnessing the colors as they began to change from orange to crimson, and then a deep, dark red-orange. As the sun approached the water, there seemed to be two suns, one in the sky and one in the water, slowly drawing toward each other.

When the sun disappeared into the water, it seemed as if every creature just stopped and admired it, making no sound that may interfere with the reverence and serenity. There was a magical stillness that pervaded everything, when the ocean was as smooth as glass and sounds seemed to be nonexistent. I so enjoyed that feeling of tranquility, and we returned several times just to witness the beauty.

Two incredible experiences together—those flawless sunsets and my first flight. I knew I wanted both to continue to be a regular part of my life.

As a child, the walls of my bedroom were covered with the planes that I was going to fly when I became old enough. Airplanes were, and still are, a passion of mine. Growing up next to an Air Force Base, an international airport, and a regional airport gave me the opportunity to see and hear all of the aircraft that would fly in and out. I could tell you about each one as it flew over, and I would dream of one day flying them. To this day, I can usually tell you the type of aircraft flying over just by the sound it makes.

As with most things in life, it all became more complicated and the days just seemed to slip by. Before I knew it, I was married and had children and my dream of flying just became one more of the things that I would dream about, but would never be able to accomplish. Or so I thought.

For my birthday in 2010, my friend, Chris, asked me if I wanted to go flying with him. He had been attending a flight school and needed to get some hours in and wanted to know if I was interested. He knew how much I loved airplanes, and the thought of actually being in the air made my enlarged heart skip a beat or two.

I answered him like I was a kid at Christmas being asked if I would like to open another present. I paced the house for hours, which felt like days, in anticipation of the flight. When he arrived, I scarcely remember leaving my family to head off to fly. That thing that only existed in my dreams was now coming true. This was the biggest dream of my life, and I still couldn't believe it was happening.

When we arrived at the airstrip, I followed Chris around, soaking in all the details of the preflight. Even the mundane task of signing out an airplane and checking the flight reports was fascinating, and I wanted to experience it all. After he had gathered his flight logs and all the necessary paperwork, we walked out into the yard and amongst the airplanes and I was in heaven.

This wasn't the first time that I had been around aircraft. Every year, the local Air Force base had an open house where thousands of spectators would come to walk around and through all the aircraft, as well as watch the world famous Thunderbirds, Red Bull Stunt pilots and other teams perform their aerial acrobatics.

I attended this every year. My son and I saw the stealth fighter the year that it was revealed to the public, as well as got an inside view of many planes, including bombers, jets and cargos. Having a father-in-law who was a supervisor on the base allowed us to see many planes that were then unknown to the public, such as the SR-71, which now sits majestically in the museum for everyone to enjoy its beauty and grace.

But this wasn't a field day at the air base where all I could do was dream of going up in one of those jets. Or a flight on a large commercial airplane that I had done hundreds of times. This was happening. I was going to fly, be in the cockpit and experience all there was to experience.

We went through the preflight checks on the aircraft, making sure that everything was operational and safe. Chris allowed me to do all the checks and walked me through the procedures. We climbed into the cockpit and my heart was ready to explode; I was hoping it wasn't a dream, but if it was, I never wanted to wake up.

After what seemed like an eternity of waiting, he finally looked at me and said, *"Are you ready for this?"* I was beyond ready; I have never been so ready for anything in my life. I was like a ball of lightning with no place to discharge.

He leaned out the side of the aircraft and hollered, *"Clear prop!"* As the engine roared to life, my heart seemed to be beating right along with the sound of the spinning prop, which in this case was about 1700 R.P.M.

It was a warm, sunny afternoon and as we taxied down the runway, I could feel the power and the exhilaration grow while we waited for our turn. As he released the break, the plane jerked forward and I realized that shortly, I would be in heaven. Except for the birth of my children, I could not imagine a day more exciting and more thrilling in my entire life.

As we started down the runway and the plane left the ground, I noticed that we just continued to fly at approximately two feet above the ground. I believed this to be normal as I was unfamiliar with taking off in a small plane. Chris and I had been friends for many years, and we knew each other very well. He is a practical jokester just like me, which is probably why we get along so well.

Chris immediately started looking around, tapping different dials and gauges and kept saying, *"There is something wrong with the plane! It won't lift."* He did this until we neared the end of the runway. This particular airfield borders a business that parks all of their semi trailers on the property right at the end of the runway, which normally isn't an issue because the runway is 4700 feet long, and the planes are already climbing by the time they get to the end.

He continued to fly right down the runway as if we were going to crash into those semi-trailers. I didn't even bat an eye at this; I wasn't concerned at all. We could have crashed and I would have died the happiest person in the world, knowing that I had flown even just that short distance. I just waited, and when he could see that I wasn't concerned, he pulled up at the last minute clearing all of the semi trailers and just laughed.

I didn't care. We were in the air. I was flying.

I just stared out of the side window as the earth drew further and further away. I watched as the buildings and cars became smaller and smaller. We gained altitude and I continued to watch out the windows of the aircraft in total awe of all of the things on the ground that honestly, I'd seen many times before from the windows of commercial aircraft, but somehow this was different and seemed to be more amazing and magical.

On this particular day, we experienced a lot of turbulence. We were flying in a small Cessna airplane, and it felt as if we were on a roller coaster. The differences in air temperature would create lifts and drops. It was never really frightening; it was just a fascinating experience to feel how the differences in thermal temperature affected a small aircraft.

We flew up over the mountain peaks, which was a view that I had never seen before. Being close enough to look down on the trees and rocks and deer; I never felt more alive than I did in the cockpit of that aircraft. We flew for several hours and upon arriving back at the airstrip, I knew that this was something that I needed to do and that flying was going to become a big part of my life.

Chris and I flew together several more times, and the majority of them were peaceful and calm. The turbulence we had during my first flight was rarely felt again; it was usually just as smooth as driving a car. We flew for enjoyment and also as transportation to and from some of my shows.

Just for fun, we would fly out over the lakes or hop the mountain peaks. Sometimes we would get lunch in other states. Pilots have what is called the $100 hamburger club. These are places that we would fly to just to buy a hamburger and it would cost us a $100 in fuel to get there and back.

Eventually, Chris started to allow me to pilot the aircraft, teaching me what I needed to know so that I could get my license. We spent hours in the air and every minute of it was a pleasure. Unfortunately, by the time I was ready to get my own pilot's license, the majority of my primary symptoms had begun. I was diagnosed with cardiomyopathy and having a heart disease that could mean a heart attack in the air disqualified me from ever obtaining my license.

This was one of the hardest things I've had to deal with. There are things that we take for granted that we may thoroughly enjoy at that moment, but fail to realize how important it is in our life. We have all heard the saying, *'It's better to have experienced something then never to experience it at all.'* I don't know that this is true because that desire, drive and need to fly is still there and I don't know that it will ever diminish.

27

THE SONG OF THE LOON

"Keep close to Nature's heart… and break clear away, once in awhile, and climb a mountain or spend a week in the woods. Wash your spirit clean."

— *John Muir*

As you may have noticed, throughout my entire life, hunting, fishing, camping and all other outdoor activities have played a significant role in the fun that I can recall with my family. As a young man, my family would spend weeks at Echo Reservoir. We would always go up over the 4th of July weekend, and would spend our time swimming, water skiing, fishing, and just sitting around the fire telling stories and making each other laugh. On the 4th of July, we would go out in the boats and watch the fireworks from the lake. It was magical to see the explosions in the sky and reflecting off the water around us. It was one of the most incredible experiences of my life, and I looked forward to it every year.

These were enjoyable times of my childhood. I learned to waterski, wakeboard and spent hours on the lake just sitting in the boat, allowing the sun to warm my skin. We'd go for rides with no particular place to go, just enjoying the wind in my face, the rocking of the boat and the scenery as we passed by.

For years, we would spend a week twice a year, at the reservoir. It didn't matter if it was bright and sunny or if it rained the entire time. Eventually the lake was privatized, so we stopped going. Every time I pass that reservoir, all of those wonderful childhood memories come flooding back.

I can still remember the sound of the crackling fire and the laughter of all of my family. The sound of the wind as it blew through the trees, the waves of the reservoir crashing on the shoreline. The sound of the boat motor, the feeling of the wind and the spray in my face as I was skiing, I didn't have any other cares in the world.

Yellowstone National Park also became one of my favorite locations to visit. My wife's family had a tradition of spending ten days there every spring on Island Park Reservoir, which is about 50 miles from the west entrance to Yellowstone Park. We would camp right on the reservoir, where we could fish and swim.

We would trek into Yellowstone where we would visit Old Faithful, Mammoth Springs and other hot pots and geysers throughout the park. On the way out, we always stopped in West Yellowstone Montana.

There were tons of little shops there that sold knick knacks and trinkets. All of the wives would spend hours going from shop to shop, looking for deals and gifts and that perfect something they just couldn't live without.

We, meaning *the guys,* knew that this was something we had to do if we wanted to fish. One day had to be sacrificed for the women. Being men, this was our logic, and we lived by it. Sacrifices had to be made. Never mind that we also found those little trinkets we couldn't live without, usually in the fly shops. We always used the excuse that we needed to find out what the fish were biting on that day.

During the summer, Yellowstone becomes a breeding ground for the Common Loon. Every morning we would wake up to the sound of the loons in the reservoir, their beautiful song echoing through the canyons. The bird and their cries become more prevalent during this season, which explains why we would hear it so frequently.

If you've never heard the noise it makes, take a minute to Google it. It's a bird that almost looks like it's wearing a tuxedo and tie. It has bright red eyes and appears to have a checker board back and pin striped neck. I know it sounds weird looking, but they're quite beautiful. The loon has an incredible sound; almost haunting, and it echoes for miles.

It is one of the most cherished sounds that I can recall. The sound of those loons every morning is a beloved memory. It is also one of the things I will miss the most when my hearing is lost.

Yellowstone was where I was taught to fly fish, and I fell in love with it. Fly fishing is an art form and it takes hours and hours of practice, but it is one of the most exhilarating and rewarding things that I have ever learned. We would go out onto the lake in float tubes, which are inner tubes with seats. We'd put on waders and fins and would paddle ourselves out into the lake suspended by the tube. We'd fly cast for trout, and would spend hours out on the lake just paddling around, catching fish.

I grew up with this. We fished all the local area's weekly during the summer, and would travel to Idaho to fish on weekends. During the winter, we would fish the rivers (minus the tubes), even though at times there would be inches of snow on the ground and parts of the river were frozen. We waded through it all just to fish.

After losing my sight, I believed my days of fly fishing rivers were behind me. Looking for just the right place to set the fly so it would drift naturally is a challenge when sighted. Watching the water break and hearing the gulp of the fish as it inhales the fly and instantly setting the hook is equally difficult. There is a great deal of timing involved with setting the hook after the fish takes the fly. In a split second, that moment has passed.

Fly casting on rivers takes great finesse and skill, too. There are usually trees or bushes that line the banks and not being able to see them makes it hard to cast without getting the line completely tangled or tripping over the natural debris lining the banks. It is a little confusing to both cast a fly and navigate the river using my cane. One of them has to go, and I guarantee it wouldn't be the fly rod.

Also realizing that, at any moment, I could fall into the rushing water and be swept down-river is a little nerve-racking, to say the least. I don't want to experience tumbling and being dragged along like all the other debris in the water. Talk about being up a small ravine flowing with fecal matter without means of propulsion.

Even with all of these deterrents, my son-in-law convinced me to try once again. I ordered a special orange fly line that was easier for me to see and I spent hours on the back lawn of my house, practicing my casting. I was a bit nervous about having the ability to place the fly in the river and not all the trees.

My son joined us, and we went to a river that I have fished many times throughout the years. I knew it to be both shallow and slow moving, but great fishing. I attempted to fish several of the open areas as we slowly made our way up the river.

I used a walking stick instead of my cane to feel my way on the uneven ground. They would tell me the direction and distance to cast, and I would give it my best effort. I honestly caught the trees and bushes almost every cast, and the few times I made it into the water weren't much better.

As the fly drifted in the current, I couldn't see if or when a fish would strike. My sons would watch, but they would lose the fly in the current or, by the time they registered a strike and told me to set the hook, it was too late and the fly would effortlessly be pulled from the water.

I eventually caught one fish and it was all of about three inches long. I haven't tried since, but I am determined to do it again.

I do, however, still fish from my tube. Most of that is fishing with nymphs, which are sub surface flies. You can feel when the fish hit those, and as long as I'm paddling around the lake, I can cast without snagging.

I always have a person there with me. We paddle along, side by side, and we talk so I can follow the voice. This remains one of my favorite ways to fish. It gives me back the freedom that I felt I lost for so long.

I still fish from a boat also, but it isn't as easy as it used to be. I'm always afraid I will lose my footing and fall. If I fall into the water, it will be difficult for me to determine which direction is up. And then there is the possibility of coming up under the boat or getting hit by the prop. All of these are issues that never crossed my mind when I was sighted.

Years ago, while earning a scouting merit badge, I had to jump into a pool while wearing a blindfold. I was confident that I could do this as long as someone was there to guide me.

The water engulfed me, and the air that I carried into the water rose to the surface in tiny little bubbles that surrounded me. As they rose, I couldn't see which way they were going. In the darkness, I was completely lost, and I couldn't tell which way to go. There was no up or down, no North, South, East or West, and I had no light to give me direction. It was like being in space, completely cut off from the world.

The object was to stop for a second, waiting for the natural buoyancy of my body to pull me to the surface. But for my whole life, I've had little luck with floating.

I can't explain it other than a theory; I had right around 4% body fat for a majority of my young life and, muscle being denser, it sinks. So when I stopped struggling to find the surface, I sunk. I should have just started swimming in the opposite direction, but I was in a bit of a panic.

I finally allowed myself to sink to the bottom and pushed off, hoping for the best. But as I emerged from the water, gasping for air after what I believed to be hours of deprivation, the second of my realizations kicked in, *"Shit, which way is it to safety?"*

This issue was solved a little faster because by this time my friends were hollering at me and I could swim for their voices. But what would I do in a situation where there were no friends to tell me which way to go to get to safety?

I have not given up swimming. I just need to be a lot more careful of where I go and with whom I'm with. But there is a solution to the boat and tube issue—I wear a life vest. I'm stubborn, not stupid.

Fishing still gives me the same thrill as it always has, whether it's from the tube or boat, or catching every tree on a river. But it's not about what I catch. In fact, one of my best friends and I have the same attitude about fishing and hunting. We spend hours on lakes and mountains with the attitude of 'it doesn't matter'. If we don't catch fish—EH! If we don't shoot anything—EH! We understand that it's the relaxation and companionship that matters.

I look back now and I realize that with all of the misery and pain my father put me through, physically and emotionally, the times we had the most fun and that I cherished, the times that everything seemed to be ok, were the times that we were hunting or fishing.

That stuck with me. That was what I looked forward to. I realize now that it was the only time my father was like a father. He still found ways to blame me, but there were times that Dad and I just sat and listened to the water flow by together, or watched the sun come up over a mountain ridge while out on the lake, and if we did catch fish, we did it together.

28

Dis-Ability

"If one can only see things according to one's own belief system, one is destined to become virtually deaf, dumb, and blind."

— *Robert Anton Wilson*

After a year of testing and hospitals, my eye specialist decided that things weren't going to change, and she made me an appointment with the counselor for the blind at the Moran. She invited me to a special 'introduction to blindness' program, to show me some of the products and services available. Some of these were extremely helpful and encouraging, but some of them didn't apply to me at all.

I found out about the Utah State Division of Services for the Blind and Visually Impaired (DSBVI), as well as vocational rehab. This was before the diagnosis and the realization that there was more to this disease than first expected. But all in all, it was a very informative and helpful process. After visiting the DSBVI and vocational rehab, I was well on my way to becoming independent once again.

Two days later, the day I had been dreading throughout this process occurred; I received my cane. I had heard stories about canes; the awkwardness and sometimes even embarrassing moments they could create. Once your cane comes out, everyone knows that you are blind. I was trying so hard to hide my blindness, but it was no use.

I was always feeling my way around, or holding on to someone's arm or even just running into things, like trucks, garbage cans, and even people. I had to accept the inevitable; I am blind, and I'm going to be so for the rest of my life.

Even now, I do everything I can to hide that fact, but overall I need the cane. When my mobility instructor arrived, we performed the 'blind guy handshake' which is basically both of us standing with our arms outreached waiting for the other to take a hold.

This is just one more thing I've had to adjust my life around. When I meet someone, I always try to be the first one to hold my hand out. That way, when the person I'm meeting sees it, they take a hold of my hand first. Which avoids the awkwardness of me trying to find theirs.

However, there are those times when I'm not first, and I miss entirely. It's like attempting to catch a swimming fish with my hand. As the two of us try to synchronize our hands, we end up chasing the other's hand around. Then there's always the missed handshake all together, where I totally miss the fact that someone has extended their hand, and I just stand there like royalty who doesn't want to touch the hand of the person who's beneath them. Or at least that's how I envision it. I'm not trying to blow people off or ignore them, but I get accused of it all the time.

After the formalities of two blind people meeting, we sat down and talked about my vision loss. This is something I've found to be quite a topic of conversation between blind people. We can all relate to what is happening, but we still have the morbid curiosity to ask the cause or onset of another's blindness.

It reminds me of the movies and stories of inmates asking each other what they're in for. They talk about all their crimes and how they got caught. We talk about the things we remember before losing our sight and the process in which it was lost.

As we got to know each other, I felt drawn to him, and I soon realized that this was going to be a typical reaction. Groups of people bond over things that they have in common; they grow and support and encourage each other. It's the same with any affliction. We all pull together to support and encourage each other. This is why groups like A.A. and N.A. work so well, and there is a love amongst them that cannot be described.

The cane was handed to me, and I felt the entire length of it. It was heavier than I thought it was going to be, and longer than I expected as well. I learned that the cane should come up to the bottom of your nose when you are standing. This allows it to be far enough in front of you to find objects such as trucks, garbage cans or people before they find you. Also, if you are walking in an area with low hanging objects, it can be held up in front of you to alert you to those items before you hit your head.

My mobility instructor spent several hours with me, teaching me the basics, but I took to that cane like a fish to water. It was like shooting a gun; it became an extension of my arm. I had one thing that I think gave me a huge advantage over others that are blind or use a cane, and that is synesthesia.

'Synesthesia is a neurological phenomenon in which stimulation of one sensory or cognitive pathway leads to automatic, involuntary experiences in a second sensory or cognitive pathway.'

The easiest way for me to describe it is *'Mixing of the Senses'*. In advanced synesthetes, most of their senses mix, meaning that they may smell colors, hear objects, see sounds or a combination of all. A permanent acid trip, so to speak. Mine is a minor case.

With my disease, it is the optic and auditory nerves that are affected, and they get mixed up. I get to see sounds. This isn't as cool as you would think, but there are advantages and some really awesome experiences because of it.

To give you an example, something as small as a dripping faucet is like an atom bomb going off every time that drop of water hits the sink. With that tiny little sound *'buopp'*, I see a giant flash of light and hear an explosion. The flash looks similar to a firework going off. One of the super large ones that light up the whole night sky and are probably a mile across.

Each sound has its own picture or light image. It could be a wavelength; if they are tightly spaced together like spikes and valleys, that would be my phone on vibrate. A light streaking across the darkness = a car horn. A combination of all three; a firework flash growing and shrinking with running lights and a wavelength = a siren on a fire truck. Everything has a unique sound, and it also has a unique pattern in my eyes.

I learned quickly that the cane as it hit the ground, a box or car gave off a different feel as well as a different sound. In no time at all, I was cruising around town, walking along busy streets and navigating malls and businesses. I have a superpower, and it's pretty amazing at times.

I spent a year going everywhere with my cane; I even used it in my house and office, even though I was familiar with these spaces, just to learn the different feels and sounds. All blind people will tell you that they see through their cane, but I truly do.

My house was also covered in bright orange tape as markers so that I could get around. We have since removed a lot of it, and I move around freely; I don't even use my cane at home any longer. I have learned my home again, and as long as no one moves any furniture, I do okay. In fact, most people don't even know I'm blind. I still have bright orange tape on my front door and some of the overhanging furniture, like shelves, because they are hard for me to remember exactly where they are.

Getting used to being disabled is not an easy task. I am constantly reminded that the term 'disabled' is not politically correct, but like everything else, it's all in the perception of the person who is disabled. It's a matter of self-worth and acceptance. I've heard 'physically challenged', but isn't that the same thing? I don't have an issue with calling myself disabled. Acceptance is the key.

I spent 40 years of my life controlling everything, and now I am dependent and reliant on others. As much as I claim to be independent, I am less so than I am comfortable with. There are many things that frustrate me, upset me, sometimes even downright piss me off. I can't speak for all disabled people, but this is how it feels for me.

First: Don't treat me like I'm made of glass! People want to help, and I understand and appreciate that, however, the *"Let me help you with that,"* to the point of actually doing it for me, is beyond helping. Except for the occasional, *"Look out, don't step there, "* or, *"Uh, sir, you're missing the urinal."* (Actually, I'm pretty happy if I'm not peeing in the sink.) All of those are acceptable and welcome. However, when you feel the need to grab my arm or shoulders and guide me through a store like a 12 year old that can't keep his hands to himself, that's where I draw the line.

Second: Don't ever say to a blind person, *"I wish you could see this."* I realize that is just a common statement, and you probably do wish I could see whatever it may be. Believe me; no one wishes more than I do. This is the hardest for me to get used to. The fireworks on the 4th of July, a deer running in a field, the sunset. But even more so, my grandchildren.

As I mentioned, two of my grandchildren were born when I was still sighted. I got to see their precious faces, the mannerisms, their smiles and tears, but I will never see them as they grow and change. Their first black eye, their first dance; never will I see them as a sighted person gets to watch their babies grow and change. I have never fully seen their faces…not like my heart wants to see them. So when you say to me, *"I wish you could see her (or him),"* that is, by far, the worst thing you could ever say to me.

Third: *"You don't look disabled."* Or, *"You're faking it."* Nothing upsets me more than being disabled and working my ass off to fit in and be independent, and then finding that people don't believe that I'm disabled. Am I just supposed to sit and do nothing and let life pass me by so that I look and act disabled? What exactly is blind supposed to look like?

I try very hard to hide my disabilities. I know that not all of us do, and it's easier for some than others. Like I said, I like being in control and I want people to see me in control. As a therapist and stage performer, eye contact is crucial. I have spent the better part of the last few years teaching myself to look at people just like a sighted person does.

I know what eye contact means for people, and I try very hard to maintain it; it's not that difficult. I have some vision, so if you are close enough to me, I know you're standing there. I may not know who you are, but I know you're there. Then I just listen to you speak. Your eyes are approximately two inches above your mouth—I listen to the words and look above the sound. Besides that, being blind opens up my other senses far beyond what I have ever experienced before.

Fourth: Don't discipline your children for being curious. Many times I have been walking with my cane and some young child will ask what it's for or why I have it. Almost immediately, a parent will stop them and simultaneously apologize to me and scold their child for embarrassing them.

This is why people are so uncomfortable around the disabled; they were taught from the time they were young that we are not supposed to ask questions or point out that someone is disabled.

HELLO, I'M THE BIG ELEPHANT IN THE ROOM WITH A LONG WHITE CANE AND DARK GLASSES! I know I'm disabled.

Two memorable experiences came from children. The first, when I was in a crowded shopping center. This, in and of itself, was a great accomplishment for me because I had very recently lost my vision and I was still trying to learn how to navigate. Being in a very crowded place only aggravated my anxieties and made me feel more confined.

As I was standing there, a small boy walked up to me and asked what my stick was for. His voice was quiet and sincere and very inquisitive. He genuinely wanted to know, and he was very polite about asking. It was at this moment that his mother stepped in and apologized to me and tried to pull her son away.

I stopped her and assured her it was okay. I then asked permission to talk to her son, which she apprehensively gave. I crouched down to his level and asked his name. *"Tommy,"* he said. *"Tommy, how old are you?"* I could tell he was looking to his mother for assurance to answer the question because there was a hesitation in his voice. He finally answered *"Four."*

"You see, Tommy, I am blind. I can't see like you or your mom. My eyes don't work anymore, so this stick is my eyes and it helps me see." At this point, I could hear the confusion in the air radiating from Tommy, but he gave me a quiet and unassured, *"Okay."* I asked permission from his mother to show him, and she stated that it would be fine, I also could tell she was now just as interested as Tommy was, if not more.

I asked Tommy to stand in front of me and hold onto my cane. I moved it back and forth so he could feel how the floor, boxes, and shelves felt when the cane struck them. I then asked him to close his eyes and imagine what each thing was as we walked through an aisle using the cane as his eyes.

When we had walked a few feet, he thanked me and went back to his mother. She also thanked me, and she was sincere and almost grateful that I didn't react the way she had assumed I would. I later learned that Tommy cheated and kept his eyes open just enough to see, but I think he got the picture.

I told you before how I was into comic books and how Iron Man was always my hero. After losing my sight, I found a new love for Daredevil. I had always read his comics, but they were like all the others—just entertainment.

Now, however, I grew a fond attachment to him and his use of his other senses beyond sight. I, too, was schooled in martial arts. I also had heightened senses and wanted to hide behind a mask.

In the series Daredevil, released in 2015 by Netflix, there is a scene where Matt Murdock is explaining how he sees. As I listened to the episode and his explanation, chills ran down my spine as I realized that is how I see as well. He talks about pressure changes, slight nuances in voice fluctuation, different sounds, and how they all come together like an impressionist painting in his head. And when asked what all of that meant he replied…

"Like the world on fire."

I replayed that over and over, and I found a higher level of love for Daredevil. He became my new hero, and I was going to do my best to mimic him. Now don't jump to conclusions; I'm not a mild-mannered attorney by day and a vigilante by night, ridding the city of crime—Well, not that you know.

The point is, as an adult, I still believe that it can all be true. Maybe not the vigilante part, but being able to find my way through other means beyond sight, having a purpose and a way to accomplish that purpose, even if that purpose is just making others believe that I am not disabled.

But back to the story, or as the comic books would say— *'Meanwhile, back in the crowded grocery department, something was about to change our hero's day.'*

I was once again standing and waiting for my escort to gather groceries and place them in the cart, because the aisles were too crowded to try to maneuver. It was easier on both of us for me to, *"Just wait here."* As I stood listening to all the sounds around me and visualizing what each was, I heard the sound of two sets of tiny footsteps approach me. They stopped right in front of me and I could hear them whispering to each other; in a sense, daring the other to speak.

I could tell that there was a boy and a girl and, judging by their voices, they couldn't have been more than five to eight years old. I also could tell the little girl was older, and she felt in charge of her younger sibling. As I stood there eavesdropping on their conversation, she finally spoke to me. Her voice was quiet and soft and very hard to discern. I couldn't tell if she was nervous, excited, curious or all three at the same time.

She said, *"Excuse me, sir."* Now one of the issues of being blind is that I don't always know when someone is talking to me. People get offended when they think I am blowing them off or have a dismissive attitude towards them, but there was no mistaking this naive girl's purpose was to talk to me.

Looking at and making eye contact with a young person is much harder than with an adult. It is tough to judge where eyes are when you are looking down. But luckily, most children are used to grownups not looking at them when they talk, so they didn't notice.

I said, *"What can I do for you?"* I was upbeat and encouraging. In a beautiful little voice, she simply asked, *"???"*

In the crowded store, and having synesthesia, and losing my hearing, I couldn't understand what she said. I crouched down to her level and said: *"I'm sorry, I didn't hear you."* Now she was much more hesitant, but once again asked in a much quieter voice, *"My brother, and I want to know if you are Daredevil?"*

That I heard, loud and clear: **"Daredevil!"**

Now don't judge me, or if you get offended, I'm apologizing right now, but these two very young people just made this blind person's existence meaningful. I hated to break their little hearts, because Daredevil is just a comic book and not real.

I looked her right in the face and, just as sincerely as I could, said, *"YES, YES I AM!"* My dream had come true, and those two little angels lit up like the orange fluorescent glow sticks. I could almost see the joy and surprise on their faces, and it made me just fill with love for my life at that moment. It was all worthwhile, feeling their joy and excitement.

I simply held my finger to my lips and said, *"Our secret."* They both nodded, at least I hope they nodded, and ran off, their day completely made by the blind man waiting for groceries.

29
Can I Get a Spot

"Sometimes even to live is an act of courage."

— Seneca

When I was young, I didn't understand the concept of 'eating healthy keeps you healthy.' My metabolism, like most active kids, made up for that. The older I got, I didn't have the metabolism to rely on as much to keep my weight in check. Even the smallest discrepancy in my eating and exercising habits added weight.

I started martial arts when I was 10, and that has kept me in shape most of my life. We used calisthenics and plyometrics as a way of training the body to be strong, but we also did weight training. The weight training wasn't to build size like the traditional bodybuilders; it was for strength.

Of course, when I was younger, my body rebuilt faster. The effects of this disease weren't as prominent. Through the process of defining the disease, I learned that most of the symptoms that would limit my abilities—heart disease, stroke-like symptoms, complete muscle failure, etc.—wouldn't come into full swing until I was closer to 40 years old.

The effects, however, were still there throughout my entire life, just in a less prominent way. I realize now that, even though I felt like I was in the best shape of my life, the disease still had a hold on me. Any physical activity seemed to drain me. I felt like I would get weak faster than everybody else and I had to fight harder to get the same distance or to push the same weight.

I know that a big part of being strong and maintaining my way of life is staying as healthy as I can. This includes eating as nutritiously as possible and going to the gym to keep my body in top physical shape. When most people think of the word gym, they automatically cringe.

They think *"Uh, sure. I'll go put forth an effort to transform myself into something I'm not, all while feeling pain and stinking up the place. Gee, that's exactly how I want to spend my day."* For me, however, the gym is a home away from home and it always has been. When I was younger and heavily into martial arts, I spent three days a week in the gym.

Later, when I was in law enforcement, I knew that if I needed to subdue someone who was larger than me, I would need that extra strength. Also, it is a psychological fact that most people won't engage in a fight with someone who is both confident and looks like they are strong.

It doesn't necessarily mean you have to be *able* to lift 300 pounds; it just has to *appear* that you can. There have been numerous times that I have seen people back down from a fight just because of the size of their opponent, even though there is no knowledge of whether they have any experience in fighting.

The gym is just as much a part of my life as hunting and fishing or being with my grandchildren. Feeling the pump and the burn after throwing weight is something I look forward to. It makes me feel whole again. It gives me the courage to take on the world, and for an hour or so each day, I can.

The gym has become my new solitude. I used to go anywhere, just my dog and me, to find solitude. Now I go to the gym. I realize this is nowhere near solitude, and I can't take my dog with me, but

CAN I GET A SPOT

I can don my headphones and be in my little world, working my body towards health every day.

I've gotten to know all of the employees at the gym fairly well; it's pretty easy to remember the blind, bald guy who walks into the gym every day. No matter who it is behind the counter, they always greet me with a *"Hey, good to see you. Glad you're back."* I always have my happy 'smart ass' remarks for them, like, *"It's good to be seen."*

When I walk in and that odor of hard work hits me, I come alive. I could be having one of the worst days of my life, but I walk over that threshold and it totally transforms. The sound and smell bring me right back to feeling healthy again. After a workout, some people complain that they're tired, but I'm just the opposite. I feel better than I do after just waking up in the morning—most days.

Another of my debilitating symptoms is called lactic acidosis. This is the buildup of lactic acid in my muscles that doesn't get removed by the same methods that everyone else has. The way I understand it is like this:

Where my disorder is an energy failure disorder related to the mitochondria, the lactic acid does not get converted back into a burnable fuel and it continues to produce and build up in my muscle tissue.

If you've ever run up a mountain side, or if you do go to the gym and work out, you will feel that tired and burning sensation in the muscles of your legs. That is the muscle tissue breaking down and the buildup of the lactic acid in the muscle. I'm not talking about the soreness you feel days after a strenuous workout. I'm talking about the burning sensation that you feel—as if your muscles are full of battery acid. The feeling of it trying to burn its way out of your body. In essence, it is full of acid, which is the byproduct of that burnable fuel.

That burning sensation in my body is created faster. It also builds to a higher level so it is more prominent and painful than for most other individuals. Lastly, it takes a much longer period for my body to process that lactic acid and convert it back into burnable fuel.

If you ever want to see a grown man cry, come with me to the gym, because I will cry real tears almost every single time from the pain in my muscles as the lactic acid builds. Without that burnable fuel, my muscles refuse to work, and that's where the energy failure comes in. Energy failure disorder fails to create the burnable fuel that my muscles need. Those muscles include my heart, lungs and every other major body function.

My muscles fail to act, so not only does going to the gym create a burning sensation, that burning sensation sometimes will last for days and even weeks. Going to the gym is not the only time that this occurs. There are many instances where I wake up in the morning in total exhaustion as if I just ran a marathon and hadn't slept all night. Although I've had hours of sleep, my body doesn't feel like it needs to move. It has absolutely no energy to rise or even get dressed.

I talked about all of the time that I have spent in hospitals in the past three years. That amount of time would add up to several months in hours, but the amount of time that I have spent entirely unable to move—bedridden—would double that. One of the hardest parts of this disorder is, plain and simple, the shutting down for four to five days at a time.

With my disease I have cardiomyopathy, meaning that my heart is weak and too large, which creates a problem with pumping blood throughout my body. It also compresses my left lung so that the amount of oxygen that my body needs is diminished.

I lose my breath rather quickly. When I lift, it's like I just got off the treadmill rather than lifted heavy weights. It takes me a long time to catch my breath. Imagine running five miles and the amount of time it takes for you to stop breathing hard after. I am always breathing hard, because it's difficult for me to get that oxygen into my system. I become light headed rather easily, and the fatigue sets in.

It is the mitochondrial DNA's job to supply energy. It's the energy production factory. Think about a steam engine, say on a train, for instance.

There's a large fire below a boiler full of water, turning it to steam. The steam is compressed, and it is used to push the train down the tracks. Using the same analogy, I have the boiler, and the fire, but there's no water. The energy that is created by the flame goes nowhere. Without compression, there's no movement. I shut down.

When I use the term 'shut down', I think of it as a machine. When the machine is running, whether it's operating at its optimum efficiency or even only partially, it's still running. If you turn the power off to the machine, it stops.

My body is just like that machine. Some days, it's working at prime efficiency; I can run, work out in my yard; play with my dogs or grandchildren. Other days, it's only working at half efficiency, where I'm able to get out of bed, get dressed and function throughout the day. But any exertion or physical activity will shut me right back down. Then there are the days when there is no energy—no power—no machine.

The only thing that I'm able to do to combat some of the lactic acidosis is take an extensive cocktail of different amino acids every day. The amino acids help rebuild my muscles faster and clear the lactic acid out a little quicker.

Amino acids are organic compounds that combine to form proteins. They are a staple in the fitness world and especially for bodybuilders. For me, it is a means of survival. I take from three to ten times the daily recommended amount, just to have the energy to function throughout the day.

None of this, however, has stopped me from being as healthy as I possibly can. I still go to the gym as many days as possible throughout the week. I work out for as long a period as I can before my body completely shuts down. I take the punishment of rebuilding and the soreness that comes with it, because without that, my body would shut down and stop. It's my way of forcing the production of energy, keeping that mitochondria working.

No matter what kind of day I have, I always try to live it to the best of my abilities. I've had to learn and face the fact that this disease is something that's bigger than me. I can't fight it like I have everything else in my life. I can't punch it into submission or debate it into conceding that it's wrong, and I'm right.

I had to learn that this particular disease needs its days. The hardest part for me is giving in when my body is telling me it needs to shut down. I have to allow it. I've come to the conclusion that if I fight it and continue to try and function throughout those days, the number of days that I shut down increases.

If I just surrender and allow the disease to run its course for those few days, my energy will return, and I can go back to my daily activities sooner. If I push through the fatigue and pain, those few days turn into weeks, and I will completely shut down and, have had to be hospitalized because the shutdown process starts to affect my heart or brain. This *'giving in'* goes completely against my nature, because I've been a fighter my whole life. I take on everything head on. Sometimes I'm too stupid to realize that I might lose. Like I said before, I'm too dumb to be afraid.

That's the truth. Being afraid is a very genuine emotion and it keeps us alive. I've had to learn that fear has its place in this disease; that I can't fight my way through this and expect to win like every other battle that I've had in my life. The way for me to overcome this is to understand it, to learn and use that knowledge to the best of my ability, rather than my will to fight.

I still fight every single day, but now in a more efficient way. I do not give up. I don't know how exactly, but the fight has changed. I have to outsmart it, out-think it, realize that when the disease is in control, I have to allow those days, so that the following days I can be in control.

I have learned many things lately; especially that I must allow my body to restore and regenerate in order to keep it strong and healthy. My way of fighting is to work my body to its limits on the days that I can, and rest it on the days that I can't. The hardest part is allowing myself to do the latter.

30

Blind Luck

"The cost of not following your heart is spending the rest of your life wishing you had.

— *Unknown*

Shooting and hunting are still a crucial part of my life. I thought for sure that would be something I would lose along with my vision. However, one of the abnormalities of my vision loss is that I can still see movement.

For whatever reason, like the fluorescent orange and fluorescent pink, I can see moving objects as well. The strange thing is that if I try and follow the movement, it stops moving and disappears. I have to stare at one spot and allow it to go through the spots in my vision. I can't tell what it is—I can't even tell you the color or shape—just that something is moving.

One of my best friends whom I have hunted with for years wasn't about to let my vision loss stop me. I was at one of my lowest points; I had started to go blind, and it was still very new to me. Mike has been there for me many times in my life and now that my vision was gone, he wasn't going to let that change. He knew he had to do something.

I received a text from him asking me if I wanted to go shooting. At first, I was extremely nervous, frightened and unsure. I didn't know if I could shoot safely. I didn't even know if I wanted to try. Generally, in sane people's minds, blind and firearms don't go together. They are two things that probably should never intersect, but it's the one thing that has always kept me alive. Mike assured me that he would be there for me to make sure nothing would go wrong and, if nothing else, just to feel the recoil of the firearm and hear the report would be therapeutic for me.

I told him I was willing to try, but I was extremely scared. He told me not to worry about anything; he would bring firearms, targets and everything else that was needed. We made plans and Mike picked me up the next afternoon.

We drove to the shooting range. With an entire mountain as a backstop, and being the only ones there, I feltl a bit better. He spent the first half hour allowing me to hold and get used to the weapons. Not being able to see them, I needed to feel how comfortably they sat in my hand. All of those memories and training came flooding back. Mike knew that I could see the color orange, so he purchased some Orange Crush in cans.

The bright cans glistened in the sunlight, and I could see them. I started to get more nervous but, at the same time, extremely excited about the prospect of possibly still being able to shoot. With an unloaded weapon, Mike stood behind me with his chest pressed up against my back; his arm stretched over mine, showing me exactly where the backstop was and where I could point the weapon safely.

He then held up one of the cans and asked me if I could see it? It wasn't the same as the bright fluorescent orange, but I could still get an idea of where it was. We loaded the gun, and we were ready for our first attempt.

As Mike threw the can up into the air, his chest was still pressed against my back, and I could feel his arm as it swung up, releasing the can into the air. As this happened, I caught a small glimpse of the can as it left his hand and by some miracle, in my mind I formed a picture of the can's flight. Almost like a drafting pencil on blueprints, my brain formulated the trajectory and velocity of the can for me.

It was as if it was being drawn in my mind; although I could not see it, it was there. Somehow, I knew exactly where the can was. I raised the firearm thinking to myself the can will be right, *'THERE,'* and squeezed the trigger.

The gun bucked in my hand, the crack of it detonating in my ears, and then silence. Mike didn't say anything; he didn't react at all, he just stood there. It was as if he was just frozen there like a statue. I couldn't take it anymore; I was ready to explode like the bullet that just left the gun. I lowered the firearm so that it would be pointed at the ground and waited, but still nothing.

My heart was beating so hard that I believe it could have broken a rib in my chest. I had no idea what had just happened, other than I had discharged a firearm. Finally, after what felt like years, I asked, *"Did I hit it?"* Mike immediately gave me a big bear hug, broke out in laughter. *"Not only did you get it, but it is dead center."*

He cleared the firearm making it safe and then retrieved the can. He handed it to me, and I felt the destruction and how well placed the shot was. I held the can in my hands, rolling it over and over, feeling all the sharp edges and how much of the can had been opened from the impact of the shot.

I put my fingers into the hole that tore through the can, feeling every inch of it. I'd done this many times in the past; somebody would throw a target up, and I would shoot it out of the air. But the feel of this can, with the knowledge that I had done this, today, almost entirely blind, was such an amazing feeling.

My emotions were all over the place; I was excited, happy, bewildered and ready to cry all at the same time. We did this seven more times, and I hit eight for eight. Somehow I hit *all eight of those cans.* I cannot explain how my mind developed a way for me to understand where the target was, but I was able to make those adjustments and hit *all* of them.

My excitement was quelled when I tried shooting a stationary target with a handgun; this turned out to be a lot more difficult.

Without movement for me to see, and no sound for me to follow, all I could do was guess. I have been shooting my whole life, certified as a firearms instructor in both law enforcement and the N.R.A. for private classes. A handgun was like an extension of my arm, but now it was like an object from another world that I had no idea how to use. Once again, Mike stood behind me and sighted the gun down my arm to the target until I finally hit it.

Next was trying my luck with clay pigeons and a shotgun. Mike threw 50 clay pigeons, and I hit 38. The 12 I missed, I had no idea where they were. When people ask me how I know where to shoot, I don't have an answer for them. My ability to explain it is lost somewhere between the action and the words. What I did know, at this point, was that I *could* do it. It was possible and I wasn't going to lose the thing that I had cherished my whole life.

After the initial experience, I brought my son along. The three of us primarily worked on my stationary shooting. Trying to hit that target was almost impossible, even with a rifle scope. My son somehow developed a way of lining up the rifle just right for me. I would hold the rifle, and he would stand behind me, look down and sight it, and he would be within inches of the target. We practiced and practiced for months, until I was able to hit the target within a couple of inches from the center the majority of the time.

In the state of Utah, we have several different types of hunts. Game like ducks, geese, or upland birds such as chucker or pheasants, along with rabbits, are considered small game. You're allowed to hunt them with a general season hunting license. Turkeys and what is considered big game, such as deer and elk, require a separate permit that are given out by drawing.

The year that I lost my eyesight, I didn't apply for any big game tags, even though we had practiced for months. I thought that part of my life was over. After this experience with Mike and realizing that, somehow, I was still able to be safe with a firearm and track moving targets, I used the opportunity to hunt small game which I had a permit for.

I've always been a very ethical and conscientious hunter; if I didn't feel comfortable with a shot, no matter what may be in front of me, I wouldn't take it. Whatever animal I happened to be hunting, I wanted that animal's pain and suffering to be as minimal as possible.

I honestly wish I could say that no animal has ever gotten away from me, that I've retrieved all of the game that I've ever attempted to harvest. However, I *can* tell you that when that *is* the case, I stop hunting that season. I look at it as if I have already filled my tag for that game for the season, and I refuse to take another animal.

I've worked very hard to instill this same integrity in my family. They all understand the gravity of taking a life. I made sure that after they had taken their first animal; I sat them down and made them understand what had just happened.

I told them it wasn't an act of malice or for the joy of killing. I made sure they understood that animal was alive, and they just took it away. I also helped them see that we do not hunt just for the fun of hunting. Every animal has a purpose, and if we take its life, its purpose is food for our family.

Hunting waterfowl with my dog was also one of my passions, and I talked about how I would go down to the marshes and use that as an escape. I went to the marshes hunting waterfowl four times, which was a slow year for me. When I could see, I would go at least twice a week. Two of the four trips I never even fired a shot. This was simply because I was terrified to shoot and didn't feel comfortable with any of my shots.

The other two days out on the marsh I shot twice, and I got two ducks. This was the first time since I was a small boy that I only got two ducks in a year of hunting. But this hunting experience was the greatest of my life.

As the first duck flew over, it was similar to the Orange Crush cans that Mike threw for me. I could hear the wings, and I got just a glimpse of its flight path. That same CAD drafting design inside of my mind calculated the duck's path.

I raised my shotgun and fired. Not knowing whether or not I hit the duck, I pulled forward further and fired a second shot. As the second shot rang out, I heard, *"You got it, you got it the first shot."* I did it. It was pure luck, but I did it.

The year after I went blind, I started applying for all of the hunts that I could, both big and small game. Mike and I both drew a deer tag, and I also drew a Swan tag. I was extremely excited but also very hesitant. I needed to know that I could do this. I needed to know that this was not lost and that I could continue with something that meant so much to me. At the same time, I was also afraid that I wouldn't be able to see the deer or that I would wound a deer and not be able to retrieve it; both of which would be a failure in my eyes.

My son-in-law, Justin, decided he would come with me on the hunt, to help me locate and identify the deer. We prepared by shooting for days, and since I hunt with a muzzle loader (a single shot rifle that uses black powder and a ball that is loaded down the barrel), we also practiced reloading drills. We spent hours obtaining the equipment for me to be able to hike around and also see the deer in the best possible ways.

I learned that walking sticks that can be purchased at any sporting goods store would be equivalent to my cane in the woods. By having one in each hand, I could swing them in front of me and feel the rocks, bushes or any other obstacles in my way. Also, having one in each hand allowed me to use them for balance when I had to step over something or move branches and twigs out of my way. After two days of hiking, I was able to navigate my way through the mountainous terrain slowly but fairly easily, which was one more accomplishment for me.

Little did I know that this was going to turn into one of the most spiritual experiences I've ever had in my life. We went up three days before the opening of the hunt to scout and prepare. I'd hunted the same area for several years, but always sighted. Now I needed to learn to move around in the mountains without vision. I barely slept a wink the night before in anticipation.

BLIND LUCK

I was overcome with extreme anxiety and fear. What the hell was I thinking? What made me believe a blind man could hunt? When the morning came, we headed out to the locations where we had seen deer. There were a few mishaps with other hunters scaring away the deer that we had picked out the night before, but I was determined. I now believe that was part of a bigger plan.

We returned to our camp in the early afternoon so that we could eat and regroup to prepare for the evening hunt. As we were sitting in camp, I was shooting a pellet gun at a target just to practice my aim and the sight picture through the scope. As I was doing this, my dog, Dozer, alerted as if something was moving through camp. Justin immediately followed my dog and looked around to see if there was anything there. He came back and sat down telling us he didn't see anything.

It was becoming late afternoon, so we started getting ready to go back out. I climbed into my camp trailer and was changing my clothes and gathering up my equipment when Justin opened the door and told me to follow him and to bring my rifle.

As I walked outside, he led me across the camp and then pointed over my shoulder and asked if I could see the deer. According to him it was 50 yards, *'directly in front of me.'* Yet I could not see it at all. I waited and searched, but I couldn't find it. I told Mike if he had a clear shot to take it. I heard the report of his muzzleloader, and Justin exclaimed, *"It's down."*

We walked over to where the deer lay, my dog close behind. We were congratulating him, patting each other on the back and making exclamations of joy. By no means were we being quiet, we were very excited.

We were talking and laughing and high-fiving each other. In the midst of all this, Justin stopped and very quietly said, *"Shawn, do you want yours right now, too?"* We all froze in our tracks wondering what he was talking about. Bewildered, Mike asked, *"Is that a deer?"* Justin very calmly said, *"Turn around."* In all of that commotion, there was a deer standing ten feet behind me. Literally close enough that I could see it—well, its movement anyway.

Dozer was over with the deer and they were sniffing each other like they were old friends catching up after being away for a long time. The deer wasn't frightened and it didn't run away, it just stood there. We couldn't believe our eyes.

If you do not hunt, this may not sound like such an incredible event, so let me explain. Deer are *extremely* skittish animals—noises, smells or anything out of the ordinary causes them to flee. All of those things were in abundance here. We were standing, talking, laughing and we had dogs, all of which should have alerted that deer to run away, but it stood and looked at us.

Although I could see the deer, I couldn't see it well enough to know if it was a male or a female. My permit only allowed me to take a male or buck deer, and I wasn't sure which this was. Justin and Mike both assured me that it was a buck.

I called my dog back to my side, which should have alerted the deer, but he looked up at me as my dog came back, then he lowered his head and started to eat. I couldn't believe what was happening and neither could anybody else. We were completely dumbfounded. I realized at that moment that I hadn't even loaded my gun. As I did, I made enough noise that, again, it should have run away, but it just continued eating.

I raised my gun, resting it against a tree so that it would be as stable as possible, and I fired. I felt the recoil of the rifle against my shoulder and heard the loud report as it echoed down the canyon. A large cloud of smoke erupted from the barrel and as that smoke cleared, I waited for confirmation.

I had missed! The deer was ten feet away and I missed. I had practiced hour after hour for this moment; I was sure I was ready, and I missed. My heart sank, and I felt like I had just found another thing that I was going to lose.

How could I miss something the size of a deer, standing still, only 10 feet away? The perfect, once in a lifetime opportunity? It was almost gift wrapped for me. Then it hit me…

Standing still!

There wasn't any movement or bright color for me to see. I was overconfident that I couldn't miss at 10 feet. Once again, the deer did not run away as we all expected, it only lifted his head, looked around and walked off, like it didn't have a care in the world.

Justin followed the deer for about a hundred yards walking behind it like it was a pet. It circled the camp to the opposite side then stopped about 60 yards out of our camp. Justin returned, the two of us got into the ATV and drove to where it was standing. We climbed out of the ATV and he helped me find where the deer was standing.

This was better, because this was how we practiced, with someone helping me sight the gun. I took my time and took careful aim, making sure of the exact shot. I switched to my left hand—I am naturally right handed, but my left eye has just a bit more vision than my right—and fired. I felt the recoil of the gun once again as the huge cloud of smoke filled the air and then the giant sigh of disappointment from my son-in-law.

All that time practicing, all the time and care I put into this, and I felt so let down. Not by the hunt, but by myself. I knew I was capable, and I missed. First at 10 feet and now at 60 yards. Justin said he would verify that I missed, and see if he could pick up the trail again.

If it was hit, we didn't want to leave it, although neither of us believed this to be the case. I stood in the silence of my disappointment and wondered if this was my sign to give up. My love and life-saving hunts were over. At that moment, I heard Justin scream *"HELL YEAH!"* at the top of his lungs and started clapping.

The sound echoed through the mountains, and I believe all the way to the nearest town, which wasn't so near. He just kept repeating *"Yes, Yes, Yes!"* I yelled with a very uncertain voice, *"Is it down?"* There was a slight pause which seemed like an eternity, so I yelled, *"Don't fuck with me!"* *"Damn right it is!"* he yelled back.

I had done it. I couldn't believe it!

Through all of the pain and darkness, I had done it. I couldn't believe my ears. I wept tears of joy, and Justin even teared up a little. I needed this, and somehow it happened. It was as if the deer was sent to me, knowing that it was something I needed in my life to reassure me. He had sacrificed himself for me, and I will honor him for the rest of my days for that sacrifice.

A short while later, Justin took me out to fill the swan tag that I drew. It was the first time that year I had gone out in the duck boat, which ironically, is named, *'Blind Luck.'* We arrived at the marsh and drove the boat the half hour into the swamp. As we did, several swans were already on the pond. We scared them and they took flight.

We got to the spot that we thought would be best and started setting up the decoys—white balloons inside a white garbage bag tied shut and weighted to keep them from blowing away.

We set up the blind on the boat and waited, but we didn't have to wait long. Twenty minutes after our arrival, we had swans flying in. We were calling, and several were circling, but I couldn't see them well enough to get a shot. I was so excited because it was so rare to have them come in so quickly.

As I listened to a small flock fly overhead, Justin urgently said, *"Right here! Right here!"* Coming into the decoys was a swan, just 15 yards from the boat, and it was landing.

I could see it because it was silhouetted by the sky. I raised my shotgun and fired. Missed! Are you kidding me? Here we go again, so close I could hit it with a bat, and I missed. But some miracle took place because it just kept coming. It didn't fly away, turn or even care that it just got shot at, it was still landing. I fired a second shot, and it fell two feet from the boat.

I feel that animal also gave its life for me. Sacrificed so that I could realize that I was still capable of living and doing what I loved. Some people argue with me, but I honestly believe that they were sent to save me. And save me they did. That's one more thing that I have accomplished and overcome, realizing that I don't need my sight to do the things that I love.

31

Mr. Heat Miser

"If we had no winter, the spring would not be so pleasant: if we did not sometimes taste of adversity, prosperity would not be so welcome."

— Anne Bradstreet

I have always loved summer. Something about the sunshine and the heat always invigorated me and made me happy. My general motto used to be the hotter it is, the better it is. I'm one of those crazy idiots who loves being in 100 degree heat.

I remember many days as a child being outside in the sunshine wearing nothing but a pair of sneakers and some shorts, running around the neighborhood all summer long, not coming back indoors until the sun had gone down.

The sun and I have always had an agreement; I would defend it to anybody who didn't enjoy what it had to offer and it would shine down on me making me happy. This worked out well and I became its knight in shining armor. People would tell me how the cold was always better than the heat because you can always dress in layers to warm back up, but when it's hot, you can only take off so much to cool down.

My argument to this is, if the only reason to dress in layers when you're cold is to be warm, then why do you not enjoy being warm when it is available to you? Many of my sunny, summer days were spent lazily along the side of a river or lake, sometimes fishing or swimming, but always enjoying the warm summer sun and heat.

Even some of the most mundane tasks which many hate, I love, because I love the sun. I loved my flower gardens, my rock garden, mowing my lawn and trimming my trees. I usually spent from the time the sun came up until it went down bonding with it even tighter.

I have also always tanned very quickly, giving me that olive colored skin. I didn't burn or peel that much as a child and I believe it was because of our relationship; it took care of me and I took care of it.

I loved going to Las Vegas in July or August. I would go there with a friend every year for a conference. We would spend a vast amount of the time out by the pool or just walking around the strip, not inside the air conditioned casinos and buildings.

At that time of year, walking in the heat of the desert sun would sentence your shoes to a slow death by submerging them into the asphalt. We would walk around in 120 degree heat like ancient gods in the deserts of Egypt. I always seemed to have more energy or desire to work and do things, the warmer it became.

My favorite pastime is watching the hummingbirds in my yard. In the early morning or late evening, just as the sun is waking or drifting off to sleep, the hummingbirds are most active. I have a particular affinity for them; they're like my spirit animal.

They remind me to appreciate life's simple pleasures and take the time to enjoy myself. This beautiful little bird is capable of incredible feats, despite its small size, even traveling great distances and flying backward.

Hummingbirds are the essence of tenacity; they have to eat three times their body weight just to sustain life. They're always vigilant in looking for new food sources. I have found this is also true in my life; I have to be ever vigilant and tenacious in all of my

MR. HEAT MISER

endeavors. I have to stay strong for the people in my life. I have to remain positive and happy.

I think about all of the trials that the hummingbird has to go through just to survive, just to maintain life. I am kind of like a large version of a hummingbird, although a lot less attractive… and I have a hard time going backward.

In some cultures, the hummingbird is a representation of reincarnated warriors who lost their lives in battle. These warriors were highly revered and therefore reincarnated as hummingbirds because of their beauty, tenacity and agility. The Chiefs would go into battle wearing hummingbird feathers around their necks, believing the spirits of the fallen warriors would protect them.

Hummingbirds are also admired as ferocious fighters and defenders of their territory. Native Americans believe that it brings luck to see a hummingbird before major events such as long hunting trips or traveling to other villages.

Watching these little brightly colored birds would create so much peace and serenity in my life. I would sit out on my deck all summer and watch them come to the feeders and show off their flight skills.

Several come back every year, and we've become trusted friends. These little guys will come up to me and chirp their song like I am part of their culture. One will sit on my head or my finger and watch over the feeder, or it will fly right up to my face and lick me as if it's greeting me with a kiss. I will even talk to them like they understand me and they chirp right back.

One summer I decided to build a new deck on the back of my home. I wanted it to be a little larger than the current one, which was more like a three-foot square landing with six stairs attached. I wanted to build a two level deck, and I spent weeks planning the look, down to the last detail, because I knew I'd be spending a lot of time there watching the birds…

I spent the next two weeks, in 100+ degree weather, building that deck. My neighbors and family were constantly trying to get me to come indoors to get out of the sun. They were afraid that I would get heat exhaustion, but I never felt more energized in my life.

Then everything changed.

Have you ever had your best friend in the world turn on you or stab you in the back? Someone that you had defended and stood up for, that you had enjoyed and played with and told your deepest secrets to, and then one day, they became your darkest enemy? This is the way I felt when I was diagnosed with this disorder. The sun had become my worst enemy, the further into the disorder that I got, the more I realized this.

As I've said, with this disorder comes a heart condition. Heat tends to exacerbate things by making it harder for my heart to pump blood. I become lightheaded, my blood thickens and less oxygen is pumped to the muscles.

On top of that, it causes me to become delirious, go into seizures, and hallucinate. Any one or a combination of these manifestations causes my anxiety to rise to unhealthy levels. The one thing that had been my best friend my whole life and that I had always loved and enjoyed, was now the one thing that caused me distress.

I have learned to adapt by completing my outdoor endeavors in the early morning hours or late in the evenings, instead of during the heat of the day because if I get too warm, I start to shut down, and I'm incapable of doing any physical labor at all. All of those beautiful summer days at the lake, camping, yard work; time spent in Las Vegas, even just sitting on my deck—are now memories.

These are the things that I look back on with joy and love, but I will likely never be able to experience fully again. It's almost as if a loved one has passed. We take for granted that they will always be there; to give advice, love, and laughter. Then suddenly, one day, they are gone. I painfully realize that the list of things I'll never experience again is getting longer. I now have to take the heat in small doses, and I have to learn that when my body starts to overheat, I need to stop or slow down and cool off.

Even as a young child, I never much cared to go play out in the cold and snow. I wasn't into building snowmen, snowball fights or

MR. HEAT MISER

sledding. I've had seasonal affective disorder (SAD) for as long as I can remember, which is a type of depression related to the changes in seasons. It affects most people in the fall and winter months, and that's exactly what I experience.

Although I did winter things with my friends or family, the entire time I was grousing. "It's going to be too cold and we're going to have to put on too many layers. We are going to get wet, and I'm going to get hungry, and I'm going to get hurt because I always get hurt," I'd complain.

I'm not saying that I never had fun in the snow. There were many times that, once we got to the sleigh riding hill or decided to build an igloo instead of a snowman, I would have a great time. But I don't look back on those as fond memories because I *did* get wet, hungry, cold and hurt, just like I expected.

Winter is harder for me now, and I dislike it even more than I did as a child. One of the things that I have always hated about winter is that it makes everything look so bland. The colors are gone, the definitions and outlines are all gone, everything appears dead and dormant.

I realize that some people get joy out of seeing the snow when it covers the trees, fences, or houses. How it looks like a sparkling white blanket and makes everything seem new and fresh. But to me, it looks like a big, white, sparkling bag of *suck*.

The only things that I find enjoyable in the winter are hunting and fishing. A lot of the late season hunting is done in the snow, and I'd get cold, wet, and hungry. As time went on and I grew older, I adjusted my hunts so they would be earlier in the year; that way I didn't get cold and wet. I also learned to take food—but I still get hurt.

Now, I'm going to throw you a curveball in here; I love ice fishing. For most of my life and, still to this day, one of my favorite ways to fish is through the ice. There's something about being in the peaceful mountain air on a frozen lake drilling a hole in the ice and enjoying the time spent fishing.

Whether I catch fish or not isn't a concern of mine, I just enjoy being there in the company of friends. In all reality, because of modern amenities being so obtainable, we take a tent and a heater and some other form of entertainment, like a radio, it's not like being miserable out in the freezing cold; it's more like fishing from a hole in the living room.

I've tried other cold weather sports, and I'm not fond of them at all, but the one sport that I've never tried is skiing. I know that sounds crazy coming from someone who grew up in Utah, with the greatest snow on earth. I have absolutely no idea what that means, but I believe it, because it's written on every single license plate in the state. People come from all over the world to ski here, and we have some of the finest ski resorts in the United States.

Just a few short miles from my home is a ski resort where many movie stars, sports athletes and other celebrities live in the winter, so that they can enjoy the skiing. But again, winter was never my friend and skiing wasn't something I wanted to do.

Now that I've lost most of my vision, navigating in the snow is even worse. The frigid conditions present new dangers and frustrations for me. Walking is a difficult task even on the best of days, because I can only recognize certain things and the ground is not one of those things.

Winter finds me flat on my back on the sidewalk or driveway, because I have slipped and fallen. I can't tell the difference between the icy surface and clean surface; it all looks the same to me. And the snow makes everything look like shades of nothingness. It's hard to explain, but what little I can see is blurry and mostly one color. Contrasting colors I can generally see, like the black top of a roadway and the cement of the curb and sidewalk.

Now that doesn't necessarily mean that I don't trip over those contrasting things. I do quite often, in fact. I can see them, but I no longer have depth perception. I can't see the height of the curbs or the depth of holes. It may look like a two-inch step to me, but in reality it's three feet.

MR. HEAT MISER

The snow takes all of that away entirely. Everything is the same color, height or depth. There are no contrasts. I can't see if there's a tree, a sign or bench in front of me because it looks the same as the background. I tend to run into and trip over more objects.

Those are not all of my issues, either. My cane gets stuck in the snow, and I get wet because I can't see the difference between the snow and the big puddle of *melted* snow that's in front of me, and you know how I feel about getting wet.

The sun reflecting off of the snow and all those little bright, shiny, sparkling diamonds of light that everybody loves so much are painful for me. My eyes try to adjust constantly to the light, but the signal never reaches my brain, and that causes significant fatigue and aching in my eyes.

Instead of little bright diamonds sparkling like Christmas lights, they turn into billions and billions of fireworks blinding me further, making it even harder to discern the differences in the path in front of me.

As much as the sun and I have always loved each other, I believe the winter hates me. I relate it to the childhood television Christmas special, *'The year without a Santa Claus' produced by Rankin/Bass*. Where two brothers, Heat Miser and Snow Miser, are always battling over seasons and territories.

I feel like I've always been best friends with Heat Miser and that made Snow Miser jealous, therefore he created more mischief and problems for me during the winter.

Ironically now, the colder I am, the better I function. I have more energy and the lactic acid that tends to build up in my muscles, slows. I have found what I would consider a miracle that gets me through each day. As I've said, as part of the disorder, I build a lot of lactic acid in my muscles, which creates intense burning and fatigue. I went from being very active and a workaholic, to struggling just to get out of bed every day.

I was introduced to a therapeutic device known as cryotherapy. This has changed my life dramatically and alleviates many of the ancillary symptoms of my disorder. Whole body cryotherapy exposes the body to temperatures of negative 175 to negative 250 degrees Fahrenheit. Temperatures this cold place your body into fight or flight mode.

Your body releases enzymes, hormones and chemicals to protect itself from the severe harm that it believes it's in. At this point, all of the blood in your body shunts to the major organs in your chest cavity, thereby pulling the toxins and acids out of your muscles and joints as the blood rapidly leaves them.

When you step out of the cryotherapy chamber and back into the heat, the veins dilate and allow the blood flow to return to the muscles, warming them back up. This is where healing and repairing begins. During this period, your body produces large numbers of white blood cells and becomes highly oxygenated.

There have been days beyond number when I was barely able to walk and almost had to crawl into the cryotherapy office. But after three short minutes in that chamber, I was ready to fight a polar bear with a flyswatter.

And now, after a roller coaster relationship, the cold has become one of my best friends; something I thought I would never say in my life. The snow is still a big, white, blurry bag of suck, but the cold gives me the closest thing to rejuvenation out there.

32

Overcome With Laughter

"You must accept the fact that there is no help but self-help. I cannot tell you how to gain freedom since freedom exists within you."

— *Bruce Lee*

At one time, I believed I would never again take pride in my yard. I had spent so many hours working on my flower gardens, landscaping and taking great care manicuring my lawn, so to feel like this was going to be lost, was overwhelming. But I took my own advice and decided not to let it go. I spent months building up the courage even to attempt the lawn mower. It's one thing to learn how to navigate a mall, but it's an entirely different prospect when you're navigating with power equipment that has the potential to sever a limb.

I mow in my bare feet, so I could feel the difference in the trimmed and long grass. The only issue came because of the three dogs I own. Walking barefoot through their land mines was not at the top of my to-do list. Talk about tiptoeing through the tulips.

I began by dragging my non-running mower across my grass. I remember one of my son's friends asked, *"Why are you pulling your lawnmower across your lawn?"* I very seriously answered, *"That's how you're supposed to do it. What do you do, push yours?"* I scoffed and continued pulling, as if he should have known that's the proper way to do it.

When I actually started the mower, I realized a few things. First, I could hear the blade cutting the grass, so I could tell if it was going over already cut grass. Also, there was a different feel as it went over long or short grass. And then I noticed that if I went in one direction and pushed the mower using it as my cane, I could continue until I hit the fence that surrounded my property or any of the other obstacles, then reverse the direction. This way I could feel the difference between the tall and cut grass and the transition from grass to cement.

It took me four and a half hours the first time I attempted to mow the entire lawn by myself, compared to when I was sighted, which took about an hour and a half. I backtracked and over mowed areas, but I did it! I was so proud and felt so accomplished; I couldn't wait to tell someone about my triumph!

Later that day, my mom came down to the house to check on me. I was so excited to show her my accomplishment, and as we stood on my deck discussing the freshly manicured lawn and I was explaining how hard it was and how I had conquered my fears, I expected to hear great praise from the one person who has always been there for me. Here's what I got:

"You missed a whole strip right there."

What? Really? Your blind son has just learned how to mow his lawn, and you're going to critique his job? She was not trying to be mean or upset me; she was just pointing it out so I could fix it. It's hilarious now!

My humor has been vital to me my entire life. I've always been the cut up—stand out—class clown. Everybody has always turned to me for humor and laughter. I've been told for most of my life how funny I am. But *I* need that laughter as much as anybody else.

I love to laugh; to be told things that are hilarious and entertaining. I love listening to other comics and laughing as much as other people enjoy it from me.

Cliché as it is, laughter is, by far, the best medicine. When this disease started, before any diagnosis or any knowledge of what was even going on with me, my comic friends gathered and did a show as a fundraiser for my medical expenses.

Some of my favorite comedians and best friends in the world showed up to perform and make people laugh. Actually, it was more of a 'Shawn Roast', as they each took turns taking a jab at me. Throughout the show, the audience responded with gasps, then you could hear them talking to each other questioning whether they should laugh at the jokes, or if it was cruel. I was in the back of the room, laughing hysterically as one of the comics on stage proudly announced, *"Shawn hasn't seen me perform in 13 years. Well, he's not seeing me perform tonight, either."* The entire room dropped to a deafening silence; you could have heard a pin drop on the carpet if it wasn't for me in the back of the room laughing honestly and genuinely.

I appreciate when people joke with me and understand that this is not my way of denying or hiding the pain. It is my way of expressing to the world that it's okay, because it's funny, and because I need to laugh.

In the iconic 1970's television series M*A*S*H*, created by Larry Gelbart; One of the characters—a psychiatrist—Dr. Sidney Freedman, was writing a letter to Sigmund Freud. As part of the letter, he wrote,

'Anger turned inward is depression, anger turned sideways is Hawkeye.'

I have always related to this statement and have replaced my name with Hawkeye's. I have taken the anger, depression and any other awful circumstance I've lived and made light of them. I used and still use my humor to get through it all; in hopes that other people can also use that humor to get through the difficult things in their life…in hopes that they can understand humor is the tie that binds us all.

It is the one thing that keeps us all going. I believe humor is the most important aspect of life. I make fun of myself—of losing my eyesight and any other circumstances that I think deserve a laugh. People ask me what it's like to go to the bathroom now that I'm blind. (It is very odd to me what people think to ask.) I tell them I go in and wander around until I see what appears to be a dark hole in the middle of white, and that's where I go. I just hope it isn't the sink.

Humor is my last respite; it's the one thing that I hope never to lose. I have had therapists and counselors tell me that I use my humor as a mechanism for hiding my fears, anxiety, hatred and depression. My reply is that I actually use my humor to keep those things from happening. It's my way of expressing my emotions; my way of telling people that it's okay, that life continues. Until I die, I will use my humor to educate, inspire and alleviate all of the tension and stress that we experience.

Even now, I perform and travel the country for speaking engagements and performing my shows. It's the one thing I still have where I feel useful and needed. Of course, it is getting harder for me to perform now; I can't see the subjects on stage or the audience and the edge of the stage blends in with the floor below. But I haven't yet fallen off the stage—I've come close, but it still hasn't happened.

I just keep moving forward. I sometimes tell everybody that I'm going to retire from doing shows altogether, then I realize that I can't be without my show. I can't be without being in front of people.

Unfortunately, it's becoming more difficult as it's now being compounded by my hearing loss. I am used to judging the success or failure of the show by the reactions of the audience, so it's harder now, since I can't see *or* hear them.

There have been shows in the past where there was so much laughter and screaming in the showroom that I couldn't even hear the music that was being played or the subject right in front of me.

OVERCOME WITH LAUGHTER

I've been told many times by many people that the laughter is just as loud as it used to be. And I still hear the laughter and know it's there, but it's not what it used to be. For me, anyway.

I realize that part of my need to perform and be on stage is a desire to feel accepted, wanted and loved. Something that I felt I never received as a child. There was a time when the greatest compliment you could give me was *"I laughed so hard my stomach hurt,"* or *"I had tears in my eyes,"* or *"I think I peed a little."*

The compliments have changed for me now. As much as I love making people laugh, it is a much greater compliment for me to hear, *"I didn't know you were blind."* or *"No one would believe you are blind."* rather than how funny the show was. To perform without the audience's pity or fear that things could go wrong is the greatest compliment I could receive.

Occasionally it can backfire. Sometimes people will approach me after the show, wanting to talk to me or shake my hand. They think I am blowing them off when, in reality, I don't even know they're there. A short while ago, a friend of mine brought her new boyfriend to my show. She was excited to introduce him to me and after my act; they came over to talk to me to tell me how funny the show was.

There was a line of people behind them wanting to express their feelings, so they hurried along so as not to take up too much time. As they walked away, her boyfriend held his hand out for me to shake and I missed it.

When this happens, and one of my assistants is standing there, they'll gently nudge my elbow, letting me know that somebody is trying to shake my hand. I felt our little signal, and I immediately held my hand out. He took it, and they left as I continued talking to others.

On their drive home, he was very hurt that I appeared to have just ignored him. He wanted me to like him because he knew how close I was with his girlfriend. He was shocked by the fact that I didn't look at him or really talk to him.

He expressed those feelings to my friend, and she explained to him, *"He's not ignoring you, he just couldn't see you. I didn't tell you, but he's blind."* He was so taken aback by this because he didn't see me as a blind person. He watched the show and had no idea that I was blind or had any other disabilities for that matter. He saw me up on that stage as every bit as capable as any sighted performer.

When I found out he thought I had blown him off, I apologized to him. He stopped me in the middle of my explanation and said how he was so impressed with how well I performed and can get around. He said he was the one that was sorry for acting the way he did. What I never told him was, that was the greatest compliment I could ever receive.

I am told all of the time what an inspiration I am. How my ability to keep going and persevere through all of this amazes people. I don't know how to react to that; I don't know how I should feel.

What goes through my mind is that they don't see me during my hard times...when my leg doesn't work, and I get angry and punch a wall. They don't see me when I'm trying so hard to see the face of my new grandchild, and all I get is blurry light and dark spots. They don't see me when I go to bed at night wondering what tomorrow may bring, or if I'll even get a tomorrow.

People only see me during the good times, during the fun. I refuse to give up and surrender to this disorder. I look out there and know there are so many people that are so much more inspiring than me. Veterans who have lost limbs and people born with debilitating diseases, still managing to live their lives. The one thing that I do wish I would have had was some forewarning that this was coming to give me some time to prepare.

I've talked to many people who have had similar types of illnesses. Whether it be Retinitis Pigmentosa, Usher Syndrome or Graves Disease; they were all diagnosed at a young age. They were allowed time to adjust and to grow with the disability. I was allowed six weeks. Six weeks. There were signs, but all of those signs were dismissed, both by doctors and me, as some other medical malady

But I am using what I have to survive, and at the top of that list is my sense of humor. I joke about what I hear, see, and experience, but as I said, sometimes people aren't sure how to respond. Their sense of humor is telling them to laugh, but do you laugh at the misfortunes of someone else?

When it comes to others and their maladies, I use my sense of humor to help them through their hard days. One of my friends recently had surgery to remove a cancerous tumor and is now going through chemotherapy. He is one of the strongest men I know, and he has a great sense of humor.

While I was going through the darkest times with this disease—pun intended—he would let me know that he was here for me in any way that I needed. Usually, that involved a jab or a punchline at my expense.

I knew these were all in fun, and it was his way of keeping my spirits up. I felt it only fair to repay his favor. After one of his chemotherapy treatments, I made it a point to send him a quick text message just to remind him I was still thinking of him. It simply said...

"I just wanted you to know that I am thinking of you and hoping all is well. Remember it's okay to cry, because if you did it would make me feel a lot less like a pussy."

His response to me was that of gratitude and laughter. He was struggling with the treatments and depression and I had made his day a little better through laughter.

Everybody has such optimism that I will regain my sight. They are always sending me links to new treatments, or ideas of what may help me. Whether it be through medication or medical procedures, everyone hopes that I will one day see again.

But no matter what happens, it's more about learning to live my life the way I am rather than dwelling on what may or may not change.

SHAWN PAULSEN

"When life isn't what you planned—make new plans."

— *Shawn Paulsen*

The late actor Christopher Reeves—a.k.a. Superman—fell off his horse during an equestrian event and suffered a spinal cord injury which left him paralyzed and in a wheelchair. He spent the remainder of his life pursuing a cure for that injury. Funding research into repairing his damage; pursuing a dream that he could once again walk.

That was his way of dealing with his loss. I am a firm believer that life is what we make it. There isn't a plan or a particular outcome. My belief is that when something like this happens, you have to take a moment and assess the situation, then ask yourself, *"Now what am I going to do?"*

I know that some people believe that God had or has a hand in my disorder. That I'm being punished for some major wrongdoing or that he will heal me. I don't want to offend anyone, but I don't see it that way at all.

I believe it is a product of life and living on a planet that has diseases as well as having a body that is prone to disease. It's not a matter of healing or finding the reason—it's a matter of moving forward with the cards I've been dealt.

I realize it's difficult for people to adjust to a disease or disorder. It's easy to become bitter and angry because you have to adapt to something that has taken away your freedom. But as I've shown, I can still be free and do the things I love even with this disease.

The majority of the money that is spent on research for any disease or disorder is devoted to those that affect the majority of the people, not the minority. My disease is so rare that less than two percent of the population is diagnosed with any form of it. It is estimated that one in three people will develop cancer during their lifetime. Research for me is far down on the list in comparison.

I am thankful for all of the things that I got to see and experience in my life. Instead of trying to get those back and spending the rest of my days in anger and depression, it's time for me to accept that this is my life now. So what am I going to do with it? I was 30 years old before I realized and made the decision that life is what I make it, and to stop waiting for somebody else to make it for me. I'm not going to take 30 more years to make that decision the second time.

I honestly believe that we're here for two reasons on this earth. The first reason is to learn everything we can, and the second is to share everything that we have learned so that others can learn everything that they can.

This disease is not a punishment; *'it is what it is.'* I'm human and humans get diseases. There isn't a plan for me; it's what I plan for me. I believe I make the decisions on where I go in my life.

I choose to take what I have, to move forward and live my life. Hunt, fish, hike, even drive. I choose to spend time with my loved ones, laughing and playing. I choose to continue my shows, performing on stage. Above all, I choose not to give up.

I don't always succeed making this decision. There are times that I am down and struggling. I do, at times, want to get out. To end it all. But I've never given up on anything in my life, and I refuse to start now.

My daughter-in-law said it best. Someone asked her how I was doing and if I was coping with all of this. She replied, *"You know Shawn—if someone tells him not to do something, he'll do it twice as hard and twice as much just to prove he can."* That's the attitude I have had with this entire disease. I'm going to show that I can do just as much just as hard as before; smiling, laughing, and joking the whole way.

33

Why Not Me

"There comes a point when you either embrace who and what you are, or condemn yourself to be miserable all of your days. There will always be people in your life who will try to make you miserable. Don't help them by doing the job yourself!"

— *Laurell K. Hamilton*

As humans, we hold within us ideas that will always be the truth to us, and they are usually what keep us in check, confirm the reason we are here and are the plan for our lives. They can be religious, spiritual, physical, emotional or mental; it really doesn't matter. And usually, no matter what kind of evidence we have, it doesn't change this core belief.

Those truths that I hold close to *my* heart are just that—*mine*. You've heard the saying that everybody has an opinion and everyone else's stinks? Well, the same goes for beliefs. People talk about how I just need to turn the page or start a new chapter or move forward in some other way. But it's not exactly about turning the page or starting a new chapter, because I believe this is an entirely new book. It isn't even the same story, with the same characters. Everything is new.

Most authors have a specific genre which they write and many of their books tend to share the same ideas. This is how my life was. It was a story with all the same characters, all the same outcomes, all the same plot lines. But once this disease took over, that all changed. It doesn't mean that it was bad or detrimental. It just means that I have a new story to tell.

I feel like I have two birthdays. The first was the day that I came into this world—June, 13 1968. The second was the day I lost my vision—May 26, 2014.

I know this sounds odd, but it really is almost like being born again. At birth, we come into the *light*. With this re-birth, it was the reverse. I came into *darkness*.

My life has changed entirely.

I know that I'm talking about my life in the past tense, as if it is over. And in a way, this is true. I've decided that part of my life is over. That book is now finished and closed.

It doesn't mean I can't open the cover and reread it. Remembering all of the experiences of the past, living all of those wonderful times once again, just like any other story.

My new life is completely different from my old life. A new author has taken over my story. The life that I live now is just as significant and just as valuable as the life I used to live. I realize that I can never go back to the things that I had when I had vision, but I definitely can go forward.

I now see things the way I remember them. Recently my wife was talking to me about an individual who works with her. I had seen her many times in her office and had interactions with her outside of the office, as well. My wife mentioned to me that this friend was going to cut her hair because it was all the way down to her waist. I immediately stopped, frozen in my tracks, because in my mind, her hair was just past her shoulders.

That was the last I saw her, so it was what I still envisioned.

That's how I see my grandchildren, too—the way I remember them. Sadly, for those who haven't been born yet or were born after I started to lose my vision, I don't have that to fall back on. For a long time, I was heartbroken by that fact. I was depressed because I believed I would miss seeing them live and grow.

However, I've come to realize that I *will* be able to see it. I may not use my eyes, and it may not be the vision that everybody else has, but I will be there. In one way or another, I'm determined that I will be there. I realize that a terminal illness makes it difficult to make that kind of promise, but I spend every hour that I can with those children; playing, teaching and loving them.

It's very important to me to know that if my life does come to an end, they will remember who their Papa Shawn was. That some of my beliefs carry on with them, and their lives are better because of our time together. It doesn't matter what I can or can't see. The bond, the emotional contact, the time—those are so much more important.

Yes, it's a whole new story from a whole new book. I'll take the new story and run with it. Make my life the best that I possibly can. It's not finding a cure or a fix that I look forward to. It's living with the disease and figuring out what I *can* do.

I have learned so much in the short few years since my second birth. I have been hunting and fishing, with great success. I have learned how to navigate through malls and city streets. I've performed in front of numerous crowds, who never knew I was disabled. I cook and prepare meals and I take great care of my yard. And I have wonderful relationships with my entire family.

I remember when I was younger, feeling so sorry for all of the people who had any terminal or debilitating illness. That they couldn't live a life like mine. Even though my life was full of turmoil, it was still great in so many ways. I actually felt pity for them, the same way a lot of people do as they look at *me* now.

Countless times I have been told it isn't fair—that one man shouldn't have to go through all of this. But I believe that this is life, and there is no such thing as fair when describing it. Fair is a word that describes gatherings in states and counties in the early fall, where people show off quilts and livestock, ride carnival rides and go to the petting zoo.

What is fair? Fair describes equally sharing something with a friend, or playing sports or how you should take a test in school. Fair is not a description of life. Is it fair that there are starving children? Is it fair that there are people who die before their time? Is it fair that people look at me as if I'm not capable of living a full life? Because isn't that what they're saying? *"It's just not fair that you can't live a life like mine?"*

It isn't a question of fair or not; it's a question of life. Life is what we make it. It's taking what we have and making the best of it. I tell people all the time, *"Life is like a poker game; you can play the cards you're dealt, or you can fold."* Folding is giving up, conceding that it's just too hard. Playing the hand you're dealt? Now *that's* the fun part. It's not even about winning the game; it's about how well you play. Yes, life is what we make it, and we need to live for every moment that it gives us, and not take a single second for granted.

I have told my loved ones over and over that they have the hardest part of this disease. They have to watch it take over, control me and, at times, completely consume my entire life. My heart aches daily as my loved ones look at me in pure helplessness, seeing the progression from day to day, knowing that there's nothing they can do.

But I am not powerless. I can live my life to the best of my ability. Keep smiling, laughing, joking and doing the things that I love to do. I can keep my head up so that they can keep theirs up. I will gladly take the burden of this disease if it means I will not have to watch my children bear it…or if I can help someone else through their life struggles.

I have heard all too many times, *"Why you?"*

My only answer is:

"Why not me?"

About The Author

Shawn Paulsen has spent the better part of his life following his passion for inspiring and motivating others to overcome the obstacles and negativity in their life. A writer, coach and entertainer, he has been entertaining and motivating audiences all across the country for over 15 years. As a comedic hypnotist, Shawn has performed in some of the most prestigious clubs and venues across the country, as well as working with some of the top name comedians in the business. Shawn earned his doctorate and started a successful therapy and life coaching business where he was committed to helping others reach their full potential. Shawn is also an educator, teaching from elementary through college level classes. He is the host of his own YouTube channel *Riding the Braille Trail* where he vlogs his greatest triumphs.

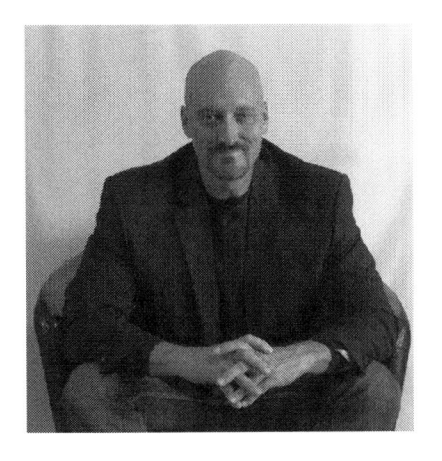

He and his wife Cindee are blessed with two children, six grandchildren, and two great-grandchildren, who are the passion of his life.

BRING SHAWN INTO YOUR COMPANY OR ORGANIZATION

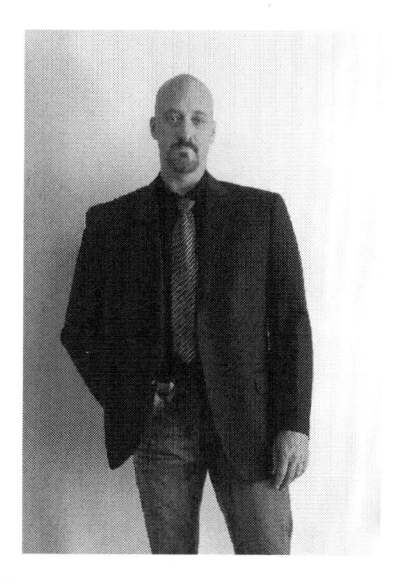

AUTHOR—SPEAKER—ENTERTAINER

With the realization that we only get one chance at this life; Shawn is determined to inspire and motivate others to overcome, and live for every moment. His hope is to show how one person's stumbling blocks can be turned into stepping stones. As a speaker, Shawn's authentic approach combined with superb content positions him as a top choice for many businesses and nonprofits.

CONTACT SHAWN TODAY:

Shawnpaulsen.com

authorshawnpaulsen@gmail.com

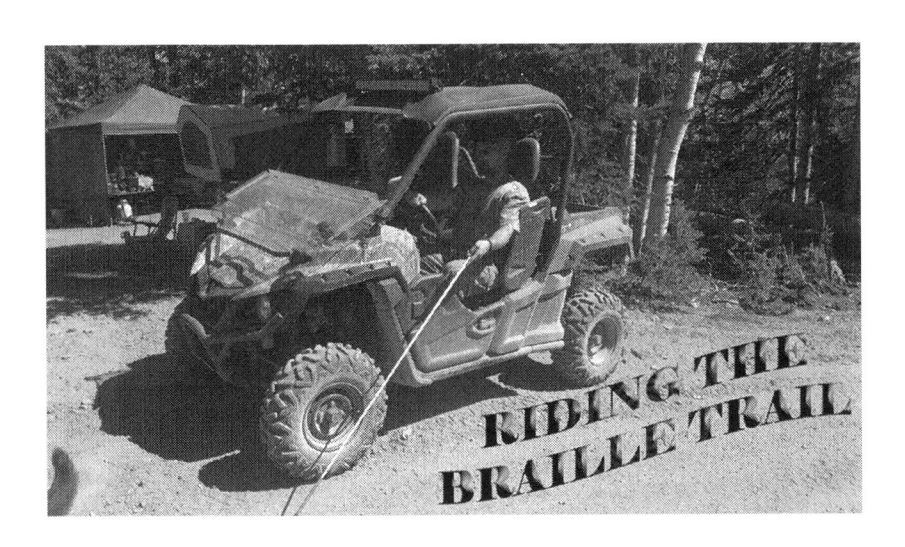

Visit my YouTube Channel to follow my newest adventures.

Made in the USA
San Bernardino, CA
25 February 2018